BIPOLAR
NO MORE

A MEMOIR OF HOPE AND RECOVERY

MICHELLE J. HOLTBY

Outskirts Press, Inc.
Denver, Colorado

Outskirts Press, Inc.
http://www.outskirtspress.com

ISBN: 978-1-4327-3138-0

Library of Congress Control Number: 2008933711

Outskirts Press and the "OP" logo are trademarks belonging to Outskirts Press, Inc.

PRINTED IN THE UNITED STATES OF AMERICA

CONTENTS

Always

To all of the caring people who have helped me in various
capacities on my journey to wellness.

Your support, prayers and encouraging words will
always be remembered.

With love, Michelle

ACKNOWLEDGMENTS

Although no one except God knows the totality of what I've been through, I'm very grateful for the people who have been in my life and who have taken this journey with me. I am a stronger person because of them. My parents—I'm grateful for everything. They gave me the physical and emotional support I needed, the space to let me sort things out, the freedom to let me become the young woman I am, their support through NAMI, and a soft place to retreat to when the rest of the world was too much for me to handle.

There's "Pete"—a shoulder to cry on and help to make sense of the world's nonsense over a good cup of Satellite coffee. "Gabby"—for our talks and neighborhood walks with Tigger. "Lori"—for our bi-monthly phone chat sessions. And thanks to all of you for encouraging and believing in me. You know who you are and how large a part you've had in my life. To Paul Coleman, your generous help sorting out music permissions (although all were way too costly to use) proved a great way to reconnect after so many years.

All of you, including my doctor, nurse, and therapist have helped me grow into the new young woman that I am. The young woman that I love. That I'm proud of. I'm thankful each day when I get up that I get the opportunity to make a difference in this world. I look forward to all of this and I wouldn't trade it for the anything.

I realize that the important thing is that I made it to the other side where I can share my story giving hope, comfort and understanding to others. I don't wish my illness on anyone, but if my book can help you in *any* way, then it will all be worth it.

"Nothing is to be feared. It is only to be understood."

–Marie Curie

THEN

MICHELLE'S SONG

There once was a girl named Michelle
Who wasn't mentally well
After 27 years
And insurmountable tears
Her life took a turn for the worse

Was it a curse? Perhaps she thought
If only I believed in God more
And kept my heart open to His door
I wouldn't go through all this pain
And for what? An endless energy drain?

Not to mention the physical and emotional stuff
That was really, really, *really* rough
That girl never gave in
What was it about her? She thought she'd committed a terrible sin
And this was God's way to get back at her

But why? And how? She wanted answers NOW!
Doctors and parents, although they tried
Could not satisfy her demanding replies
Weekly doctor visits and medications galore

Did little to answer the questions knocking at her mind's door

"Will this drug make me fat?
Gaining weight, I can't stand that.
Will I be killing brain cells and slowly losing my mind?
Please, tell me now, I don't want to be left behind."

7 years have since passed by
My oh my, how time does fly
Yet for me, it seemed to come to a standstill
God slowed things down and then gently as a whistle

He called my name in the night
And with not so much as a fright,
I sat up in bed and rubbed my eyes
And grabbed an empty journal nearby
Just waiting for me to open the first page
And write down things that were locked up in a cage.

And those very words you see
Were what was the beginning of setting me free
Bipolar disorder I did not ask for
But writing this book is exactly what God had in store.

By Michelle Holtby © 2008

INTRODUCTION

Bipolar No More is my memoir of a blessing disguised as a tragedy. It's my personal story of living with bipolar disorder.

I haven't discovered a cure, I'm not in denial and I haven't stopped taking my psychiatric medications every day. So, how can I *not* be bipolar anymore? My book unveils the answer through my journey of living with this debilitating, yet freeing illness from the time prior to my diagnosis all the way to the present day.

Mine is a story of hope and recovery. I share it so others may find comfort and understanding. No matter what the stage of their illness, recovery is possible for those afflicted with bipolar disorder.

Bipolar No More is informative, humorous, scary, insightful and thought-provoking. It has to be all those things to convey what happened to me and how I rebuilt my life after my diagnosis. Today, I accept and understand my mental illness. I've written this book to help others get to a similar place. By telling my story, I hope to get readers thinking about their own stories. People need to open up and talk with each other to break down barriers of stigma and to let in comfort, hope and understanding.

...

In May 1996 I graduated with honors from New Mexico State University in Las Cruces, New Mexico. I thought the world would open up new doors for me to explore. This was my time to make my mark on the world–to make a positive difference. I was enthusiastic, happy and free to make choices for the lifestyle I wanted to have. And earning a paycheck was definitely a nice perk.

In May 2001, at the age of 27, I was diagnosed with a mental illness also known as a brain disorder. I thought I was God. I lost everything overnight: my job, relationships, dignity and my self-esteem. It was too much to get a handle on. I couldn't comprehend any of it.

"Why, God?" I kept asking. "Why did you give me this debilitating illness that would lead me to nothing but having to start over?" I wanted answers. Unfortunately, my parents and my doctor couldn't answer all my questions, but my daily journaling helped.

I felt absolutely hopeless and numb. Tears of loss and fear steadily trickled down my face, off my chin and onto my journal pages. What I wrote spanned several years and it seemed like dumping out mental garbage. I felt like someone had played a really mean, irreversible trick on me. I wasn't a bad person. Why did this happen to me?

There is no redo or going back once you're diagnosed. There are only two choices: staying stuck or moving forward. I chose to move forward. It's been a long, slow emotionally painful process that has led me to be a stronger person.

...

Since my diagnosis of bipolar disorder more than seven

years ago, my previous life no longer exists. I now live at home with my parents and my dog, Tigger. I am a published author, as well as a freelance writer and graphic designer. I'm also involved with the National Alliance on Mental Illness (NAMI) "In Our Own Voice" (IOOV) Program.

I've been a presenter for four years and have shared my personal story of living with mental illness to people in various venues, including at the UNM Mental Health Center, where I was diagnosed and twice hospitalized. I was also the Peer Coordinator for one year, arranging presentations in the community.

Being involved with "In Our Own Voice" (IOOV) has helped me in many ways. It's been a blessing to be able to share my experiences of living with bipolar disorder with other consumers, family members, friends and the general public. It's also helping me to heal. Unfortunately, mental illness has no warning–and you won't be prepared unless you happen to know it runs in your family. And even then, it doesn't hit everyone. In my case, it even skipped a generation.

Bipolar disorder, formerly known as manic depression, affects more than two million Americans. It's a chemical imbalance in the brain that can be corrected with the proper psychiatric medications. Bipolar disorder is *not* something that can be "snapped out of." But with the help of medication, psychotherapy and support from family and friends– including support groups–it is quite manageable and a person can live a productive life.

The three types of bipolar disorder include I, II, and cyclothymic disorders. Bipolar I disorder, the focus of this book, is the most common and most severe form of the illness. Psychiatrists define bipolar I disorder as having one manic or mixed episode(s), with elated mood and three others associated symptoms of mania (grandiose thinking, such as thinking one is God), a decreased need for sleep, pressured (rapid) speech, increased activity or energy level, racing thoughts, flight of ideas, distractibility (hard to focus on anything for long periods of time or jumping between several activities in a short period of time or impulsive behavior), or shopping or spending sprees, much like how a small child acts (without consequences). These symptoms must last a week or more and require psychiatric hospitalization.

The good news is that by continuing with improved medication, those with bipolar disorder are able to function well and often experience a reduced level of side effects.

While there is no cure yet for bipolar disorder, I have hope there will be a cure within my lifetime. But, until then, I take my medications faithfully each day and follow a daily schedule that helps keep me on track and minimizes the anxiety and stress I experience.

I wrote *Bipolar No More* for three groups: for those with a mental illness; their family members and friends; and the general public. Why? To help educate, give hope and eradicate stigma. The media currently focus on mental illness in a minute portion of the mentally ill population. No one sees healthy people living with this illness. May my book enlighten people to see the other side of mental illness–the people who are highly functioning and who have families, homes and jobs.

Writing this book helped save my life. May it bring you comfort, hope and understanding.

Michelle Holtby
Albuquerque, NM
July 2008

CORPORATE AMERICA

"What doesn't kill me makes me stronger."
—Albert Camus

I am bound by a number—127 pounds. My security. My one thing I can control in my out-of-this-world insanity I am experiencing. I hate it! My world, that is. Well, fine then. No, it's not fine. It's the complete opposite of fine. It sucks! And no matter how much I rant and rave nothing's going to change. I chose this job and now I've got to live with the consequences.

Weighing myself on my digital scale each morning before getting dressed made me anxious. 127 pounds meant, "It'll be a good day," like winning the lottery or having a horoscope come true for a day. Any weight above that number altered my mood to negativity and consumed my mind all day with anxious thoughts: Why did I gain two pounds? I'm losing control. I've got to get back down to 127 pounds.

Yes, I thought, 127 is the magic number where everything is okay. I feel presentable and accepted by my co-workers. I feel sure of myself (sigh). But can people tell what I'm thinking?

My thoughts taunted me: Look at me. This is what you

1

wanted. Your robot is now the size and shape you wanted. I was dead inside and I had no thought of my body other than it was a shell to showcase to the world—a mannequin that was hollow, dark and lonely. But no one could know this from the outside, could they?

Every morning upon entering the "door of doom" (my place of employment), I took a breath and put on a smile I hoped would come across as my being pleased to be there. I faked my way through each day, convincing even myself that I loved my job and that my co-workers liked me, as well. That couldn't have been any farther from the truth.

My clients were what kept me going, especially the ones that reciprocated my caring manner, which was totally genuine. And they gave me hope. I felt safe to let down my Corporate America guard and just be me. That is why I spent a considerable amount of time outside the office. Traveling around the state allowed me freedom, space and time to think.

"Toxic city" was slowly killing me and my spirit. It was a slow death—2 ½ years in the making. But the one thing Corporate America was unable to chop to pieces, like a culinary student still learning knife tricks, was my creativity. My thinking outside the box and creating billboard advertisements for my clients was what I enjoyed most. Unfortunately, the dinosaur demolishers (management) were not supportive of that.

I didn't care if I was rocking the boat. Since I was a child, I never fit in a box, so why start now? I felt free to express myself in the presence of my clients. Being able to create advertisements with my clients was like putting a puzzle together, one piece at a time. I slowly and gradually gathered information from their companies to create simple and effective advertisements designed to produce business and keep them renewing their contracts with me. And that would help me keep my job, although for some unknown reason, I thought I was going to get fired from day one.

I was my own boss when I was creating ads. No parameters to follow. Absolutely nothing to stop my creative juices from flowing from my brain onto my paper. I'd smile and think: This is a really cool idea. I can't wait to share it with the other sales people at our staff meeting. And I looked forward to brainstorming with them to get additional ideas.

After about a year I came to the realization that no matter what I designed, it would get shot down in one way or another. So much for a supportive boss and sales team. Honestly, I got more support from my bra than I did from my co-workers.

The lack of support and encouragement from my boss and co-workers was a huge disappointment. I'd try not to show it though, when I walked into my boss' office to share what I'd created, only to receive criticism.

I was surprised because I just sat there taking it. I didn't understand why she was diminishing my creation to the size of a pellet in a wood burning stove, and I didn't know what to say. I wasn't expecting the conversation to go like that at all. I think I remembered to blink, though. I was stuck to my chair with disappointment that weighed me down so much I couldn't budge.

The receptionist's voice startled me. "Mr. Jones is on line one. It's about his ad." Whew! Thank goodness for the rescue from yet another upset advertiser wondering why their ad hadn't been posted yet.

That was the story of my life when I worked for that company. *Everything* was an emergency. You'd think people were going in for bypass surgery with the amount of urgency inflected by the tone of their voice on the phone.

I said to my boss, "Your client's call sounds urgent. I'll let you get that." I left her office thinking, you know, people, this is not an emergency room. Yes, you may think the end of the world is coming if your advertisement doesn't get up, but here's a news flash: IT'S NOT! Oh, how I would have loved to scream that statement to them over the phone, but I maintained my composure by banging my head on my desk a few times— when no one was looking, of course.

Sometimes I'd just stare at the phone receiver and won-der what planet some of these clients were on and if, by chance, their priorities were a bit off kilter. Then when I had hung up, I'd bang the phone on my desk to be rid of excess anger at their impatience and stupidity. If that didn't suffice, then I'd bang my head on my desk a few times. Why, oh why, God, am I here? Is this what my life has amounted to? Talking with people who have no perspective on life? I hate this, I whispered, while choking back tears. I don't know how much longer I can go on. I'm not like them. Please help me. Please. Someone.

Some of my clients amazed me and not always in good ways. I'd say I ran on pure adrenaline six of my eight-hour days. This did nothing to calm my nerves, to allow me to breathe before diving deep into my next client's file. With busy work, returning calls, sales meetings, visiting clients and walking around the office with a pleasant grin on my young face, I felt like a puppet.

Go ahead. Tug this string. What will it do, my co-workers pondered? Oh no, she's crying. Wait. Okay, let's try again. Then they pulled another string and waited.

"Yes, Ms. Jones," I said. "I have your contract. I'll be over at 2 PM today. Yes, it looks great. See you soon. Bye."

"Whew! Amazing," my co-workers said. "She's able to say all that in one breath. No wonder she's so productive."

One employee inquired, "What drug are you on, dear?"

"No drugs," I replied. "Just pure adrenaline and the willingness to please my client's needs as fast and accurately as possible. Making the sale. That's what it's all about. I'm better than Wite-Out, baby. I don't make mistakes and the best part is I don't stink or leave fumes like that little bottle does. So, move out of my way. I'm plowing through."

I'm surprised I didn't completely wear out the soles of my dress shoes. Faster, faster, leaving a trail of perfume behind. Swish, swish. Note: Always be sure to wear pants or soft flowing skirts to allow for optimum walking speed.

One-half-inch heels were my maximum shoe height. Flats were preferred. I could almost run in them to get to the fax machine to send a copy of a contract to a customer. Yeah, if it wasn't for the tile floor I would have had *much* better speed. If only I could have found dress shoes with rubber soles. Unfortunately, tennis shoes weren't encouraged.

Change is good. Oh, no. Wait! They don't like thinking outside the box. So, maybe a toboggan or, better yet, tubes set in the ceiling, like at the bank, to transfer information back and forth quickly with no physical exertion.

That was how I stayed in shape: walking about a mile each day from my desk in the back of the building to the supply office. And if I walked fast enough I could avoid being stopped by other co-workers wanting something from me. Leave a note on my desk, I thought. A voicemail will do. But, get out of my way because I'll plow you over, otherwise.

I was utterly stressed and miserable—all for a paycheck. I'd drive home every day from work and cry for hours. I thought this was what all successful people did. And no one would talk about it. They'd just wake up the next morning and do it all over again.

I decided that if I was to survive in this God-awful job

I'd better do *something* to protect myself. So, bye-bye former happy, carefree, easy-going, fun, laughing, college-days Michelle. And just like that, I snapped my fingers, looked in the mirror and made an oath.

To this day, I make promises to myself I still stick to, as I did with that oath: Michelle, girlfriend, it's time for you to wake up and see things for how they are and not how you'd like them to be. You can only change you—not others. How others treat you is none of your business. Your goal is to survive in this land of bullshit Corporate America. I vow, from this day forward (September 20, 1996), to protect myself in all ways possible. I will arm myself with a full-body invisible shield that will bounce off negativity from others. I will surround my home and office with images of creativity, inspiration and love, and I will remain in the office as little as possible to preserve the small amount of energy I have left to go and meet with clients.

It was quite an oath—but one that worked. Sort of. Me, the planner that I am, didn't allow for quirks or uncontrollable things to pop up—things that threw me off course, denting my daily routine that my new "corporate" body was just getting used to. I felt like a Ping Pong ball being whacked hard, side-to-side, at a dizzying rate. And I felt on the verge of having a nervous breakdown.

I wondered, would this be a record at age 22? I was so overstressed and under-appreciated it amazes me now how I was able to keep it all together, at all. But, like I said, after 5 PM, like clockwork, the hot, stinging tears burning with rage would start rolling down my cheeks. "It's not supposed to be this way! This is not what I went to college for!" I screamed behind rolled-up windows as I strangled my steering wheel like Hulk Hogan.

I wanted out, but I feared the consequences. I wanted someone or something to console me. And that became my television, my 5–10 PM reliable friend, five nights a week, which blocked out my sorrows, worries and made my mind go numb from the day. It put my thoughts to sleep, but kept me up all night tossing and turning with nightmares of being fired, co-workers talking behind my back and finding ways to retaliate and gang up on me.

Unfortunately, my over-creative mind would often take me to places that left me paralyzed with fear and overwhelmed. Every morning, I raged inside, "I didn't go to college for this. I want my old life back. I can't do this anymore. It's much too much and it's not me. I hate me. I truly hate who I am at work because it's only a façade.

"Putting on a plastic face," I called it. You gotta' look happy and confident every day, no matter how crappy you feel, so you can go out in the world and earn your salary. I just wanted to die. I was already completely dead inside. I had no life. This is not living, I thought, it's merely surviving. It's treading water just enough to keep my head above it every damn day.

I was hoping *someone,* on an emotional and physical level, would recognize my cry for help and, like bobbing for apples, would pull me up out of the water, dry me off and be my friend.

That was another thing. I had no friends. I had a few acquaintances at work, but I was the one left out of many functions because I was young and single—two strikes against me. I didn't know then that age and marital status determined your peer-acceptance rate and level of being included.

Who am I kidding? I thought. I'm a freshly grown college graduate with a world of enthusiasm, creativity and enough energy to hit the ground running. Oh, they let me run all right, on the never-ending treadmill that eventually landed me smack dab up against a stone-cold cylinder wall, leaving nothing but an outline of a young woman who had been so full of optimism, ideas and spunk.

So, the question remains, if one's creativity is stifled, ignored, laughed at or stolen in the world of advertising, how does the company make any profit? Doesn't seem like rocket science to me that encouraging someone's personal growth, encouraging them to think outside the box and brainstorm, and avoid stealing other ideas would be such a bad thing.

I'd say having this realization at age 23 would probably not quite fit into the box of nominating myself as CEO of the company, but I would have considered being a manager.

What a bunch of mentally and physically disorganized monkeys—I mean people—who surrounded me during our weekly sales meetings. And how I dreaded those damn meetings. Issues were discussed using a pecking order based on age and years with the company, with the most important and current "crisis" on the table.

I had such high hopes of one day filling their shoes— NOT! It was all a bunch of crap. And for what? A pretty little paycheck tied with a bow, like being handed a diploma, only you never graduate. You do it all over again every Monday morning—the day when the treadmill of stress starts taking its toll for another new week.

Step right up. You, too, can be a sucker in life who sells his soul to achieve the American Dream: a big house, married with two kids, an SUV, a boat and numerous debts, which is why you have to keep running on that treadmill.

Occasionally those monkeys *did* make me laugh—at them—but not with them. Sometimes the laughs came from their ideas, but more frequently, just from observing them. By mostly listening. Gradually, I adapted some of their techniques into my phone conversations with my unique clients and presentations. I actually dropped my guard a little when I was at my desk creating an ad. I loved what I came up with, but rarely showed my work to anyone prior to approval from my client.

It took almost a year of personal and professional growth, plus one more year tacked on the big "22" to finally feel—in the spring of 1997—like I was getting the swing of how the company worked and whom I could trust. That and some other things continued to lower my armored barrier. I was learning to like myself again and I didn't go home crying anymore.

Things seemed lighter, easier. I laughed more and my carefree attitude returned. It reminded me exactly how I felt during my senior year at NMSU. I felt like I'd reclaimed my college years and I was now at a point where I could pick up where I left off—and earn a paycheck, too.

This easy, laid-back version of me continued through the summer. I had an easier time relating and talking to co-workers, when not feeling the initial exclusion and judgment of the prior year. It was as if all the hatred, sadness and resentment since I was hired in July 1996 were forgiven by all.

I loved being me. I enjoyed going into work each morning. I talked with co-workers and clients with ease, trust and confidence. I don't know if others noticed a change in me, but more importantly, *I* noticed a vast change in me. The "me" I thought I had lost after graduation returned— and just in time. I had begun to lose hope in all areas of my life. But I felt as if God were looking out for me and had picked me up carefully and helped me to get back on track. I had just *thought* I'd really gotten off-track, which was why I was so miserable. But now, God rescued me and placed me back on track. Things were easier again. And they were—until fall, 1998.

• • •

For no apparent reason, my mood changed overnight as if switching off a light. In trying to analyze it, I couldn't pinpoint any one thing in particular that had occurred the previous day to change my mood from sunny and carefree to gloomy and irritated.

I got up and went to work, feeling as if I were having a bad or "off" Monday—only it was Thursday. I went through several days with the same gloomy, gray cloud of irritation and sluggishness. I never mentioned how I felt to anyone. I thought it was merely my personality, but the gloom lasted until the following spring.

My parents, doctor and friends said nothing. They weren't around me for a long enough time to see the obvious personality change I'd undergone.

• • •

To say the least, my feelings did nothing to help me keep my job. Each day I dreaded going to the office. After tossing and turning all night I could barely drag myself out of bed. Waking up each morning feeling anxious and overwhelmed were normal feelings for me while I got ready. With growing dread I drove closer towards my office building every day. Damn I hate this place, I thought. I know I'm good at what I do. My clients like me, why don't my co-workers?

Feelings of resentment and retaliation came back to life that fall of 1998 and lasted until the spring of 1999—what seemed like an eternity.

Someone switched the light on again and, as if being awakened from a bear's long winter slumber, I became my happy, carefree self again. Man, I loved that time of year.

But I felt *too* alive. I was easily able to talk with others, I created and I had unflagging energy that often kept me up late at night while thinking and creating new projects as a way to release all of my pent-up energy.

I would literally run over people at work, deeming that my clients were of the utmost importance. Zipping up and down the hallway, I sent faxes, made phone calls and checked production—all at warp speed. I didn't need to join a gym. I was busy burning rubber racing through the hallway most of the day. I felt completely in control, although it was dizzying, at times.

Got to accomplish this today, send a fax to so-and-so, call two clients about updates on production, blah, blah, blah, I thought before I even entered the office. Never mind a Palm Pilot—my mind was geared into overdrive, and I was flying on pure adrenaline. I totally loved it. I thrived on it. No caffeine kick was needed. I was the most efficient, organized, successful salesperson that season—and my paycheck proved it!

But it wasn't the money that drove my energy level; it was always the next sale. Always another fish out there to catch. How long would it take me? Could I beat the competition? My self-motivation pushed me physically and mentally. Did it take a toll on me?

Well, at age 25, I was fortunate enough to be fairly resilient to physical ailments. It was the compounding daily stress that my body wasn't coping well with. My insides were being shaken up and my body reacted by exerting excess energy, sleeping less, creating more and talking faster. These were all things that I loved about myself and without realizing it, they were gradually escalating as each season passed.

•••

After two-and-a-half years of working in that advertising job, I got bored. I felt I'd outgrown the position. And I wasn't being challenged enough to keep up with my highs. So, somewhat spontaneously, I decided to change jobs and choose something completely different—financial planning. Me, who took an entire year at NMSU to pass algebra with a C. (Guess I'd conveniently forgotten that.) But I had gotten an A in my accounting class, so off I went to my money management career.

My boss and I got along well. Through various connections, she had heard I was looking for a change, and she was interested in hiring another consultant. Timing is a beautiful thing. With two months remaining at my advertising job, my mind was dreaming ahead, thinking about a straight salary (bye-bye commissions). So sad—NOT!

I was looking forward to a small office, casual dress code, and getting along with the other workers. Yes, I was walking around my last two months in Corporate America wearing my advertising face, only it wasn't fake. I felt so elated I was like a balloon floating toward the ceiling. Light and happy and free. Yes, I was soon to be set free from what I had once thought was going to be the start of a wonderful, exciting career in advertising.

I was a bright yellow balloon to begin with. But my initial enthusiasm and great ideas, optimism, (not to mention a college degree) and knowledge were slowly deflated over those two-and-a-half years until all that was left was a flat balloon on the floor—stepped on and stuck with gum.

It's sad how some people don't recognize talent even when it's right in their face. Not to bother, though, I thought. I was going to peel my yellow-balloon self off the advertising world floor, clean it up a little, maybe draw a smiley face on it and start over.

Some lessons in life were disappointing, unfair, or, in

this case, just plain sucked. But the best part is they didn't take away my creativity (a wonderful bipolar result), my sense of helping people and my wonderful clients whom I got to know as people—some even as family. I've always enjoyed helping others, especially finding matches for people. I like putting puzzle pieces together.

I had no regrets leaving the advertising job. I learned what I needed to learn and no matter how unpleasant the lesson, I did grow from it. Unfortunately with the growth came the introduction of putting up a wall towards everyone: not trusting others, avoiding people and finally leaving the office. Damn, I hated it there half of every year from September to February. If it hadn't been for my rent payment I would've bailed out much earlier.

Beginning in January 1999, I worked for a family-owned business that was definitely a welcome change from having to chase after clients. The whole commission thing was definitely not missed. From 8 to 5 PM, Monday through Friday, I sat at a desk, talked to clients on the phone and prepared financial reports and statements. I picked up on it pretty quickly. I enjoyed the work, and it was a comfortable pace for me. No sales quota to meet. Precision was key. And details and thoroughness were and are two of my strong skills.

I was enjoying learning about the business and really liked the fact there were only six of us in the office, sharing two rooms. My paranoia and feelings of being overwhelmed were tucked to sleep in the back of my brain and I was able to focus and make suggestions to clients. My boss trusted me to make decisions, which was great. I've never done well with a boss standing behind me, watching and listening to my every word and movement.

I've always enjoyed the newness of a job. There's so much to learn and discover. I find it fascinating, probably because I'm a very curious woman. I like to know the "why" and "how" of things. And I fed off this fact. My brain was like a sponge, hungry for more knowledge. The more I learned, the more I wanted to learn. I think that was why Cindy, my boss, had such confidence in me and trusted me to recommend things to clients that would help their business grow.

Being very patient, knowledgeable and thorough were a good combination of skills for the job. It was up to me to pace myself each day. Setting my own schedule was great. At the time, I felt no bipolar symptoms—everything was okay with my emotions (no crying spells or elated energy). I definitely liked being in control, so setting my own schedule, working with clients to create and modify their budgets, preparing financial statements and making recommendations on how best to allocate their money was a wonderful confidence booster for me. But to have trust from my boss—that was a welcome first.

•••

Things moved along smoothly for the first year. One of the consultants left and a new woman was hired a few months later. It was pretty quiet. Oftentimes I worked alone in the office. It didn't bother me. I'd turn on the radio, sing along karaoke-style and sometimes I'd dance around to a good song while I worked away.

During the summer, things quieted down—a seasonal trend—so I'd get to go home early. Man, this is cool, I thought. But the times I was working alone I'd think: So this is what it feels like to own your own business? I could definitely get used to this.

I really thrived in that environment (I now realize that), just enjoying it for what it was and for however long it would last.

Sometimes my boss would call in sick, or leave for vacation or had company coming into town, and she'd ask if I would mind taking care of things in the office. I was always elated when I got these calls from her (dance of joy, dance of joy). Oh, of course, get well soon, if you're sick, but yeah, baby, just me, the radio, the scenic view out my window and peace and quiet.

The first year working for Cindy was fine. Why can't things remain status quo for me in the world of work?

In year two things started getting weird (rather, Cindy got weird and I got pissed off). Turned out her phone calls into the office explaining her excuses for not coming to the office weren't exactly truthful. As a matter of fact, they weren't the truth at all.

In the fall, business began to pick up for the upcoming season and I began to see Cindy's happy face, nicely dressed, hair and makeup on—suddenly gone. Like overnight. I remember (this is engrained in my mind, it was *that* bad) her walking into the office on a Monday morning, with her hair in disarray (like she'd stuck her finger in a light switch), carrying the morning paper under her arm, along with a bag of gourmet coffee beans. She had just thrown on a shirt and shorts, and did not look like she had showered. But the most noticeable "wow" thing that caught my eyes was that she was wearing sunglasses.

I didn't say anything. I just watched "it" gravitate towards her office. All I can say is thank goodness we didn't share an office because I would've passed out from her foul odor. The smell was on her breath—alcohol. Damn. I can *still* imagine the smell.

Bourbon? Scotch? I don't know. I was a wine cooler drinker, myself. But whatever it was, it was strong and—at that moment—the connection suddenly came together for me: her calling in so often during the summer, looking and smelling like hell and wearing sunglasses.

I guess her one saving grace was her bag of coffee beans. I offered to get it ready for her. I did have compassion for her, even though I didn't understand or know that side of her. It sort of frightened me. I'd never been exposed to an alcoholic in all of my 25 years. Guess I was lucky.

Still, I didn't think I was going to have any luck heading down to the local library to research "alcoholic supervisors and how to cope with them in the workplace." I didn't even bother to make the trip to the library. I figured she'd had a party over the weekend and this was the end result of it.

Cindy's coffee finally kicked in about noon. She removed her sunglasses, raised her window shades and emerged from her office pretty much her usual self. We talked for a while. I worked a bit, then she let me go home early (I thought it was probably consolation for her morning greeting). Well, tomorrow would be a new day, I thought. And I enjoyed getting off early. I went to get some ice cream, rented a video and headed home to spend some quality time with Tigger.

Have you ever seen the movie, *Groundhog Day*? How every day, everything happens at the exact time and exactly the same way as the day before? It's a rerun, with no changes.

Welcome to day two, through day 180 when I resigned six months later, thinking, how dare she contaminate my work environment? My peace and enjoyment. Damn witch! Great, here goes my bright yellow balloon being deflated again, only this time it only took one pristine, shiny dart to deflate me.

The only problem was I had no back-up plan, no lead. Great. What am I going to do for employment now? I thought. There was more at stake: a mortgage payment. Okay, I can do this.

Fortunately for me, Cindy was coming into the office later each morning, so for those first few hours, I spent my time on the internet looking for my next job. Honestly, I wasn't too particular. I just wanted—correction—I *needed* to get out of there and fast. Mayday, mayday, this ship is going down fast and I'll be damned to die aboard it.

I had the same focus and energy and, fortunately, enough time to research potential companies. I don't remember how long it took me to find an answer to my prayers, but one came and I snatched at the opportunity, working in sales, for a radio station. Okay, is this a sign or what?

In January 2001 I began job attempt number three by selling radio advertising for a local station. Once again, the cycle began. I was really excited (and thankful) my prayers had been answered. Okay, if I could generate the sales numbers to keep my boss happy, I thought, this might turn out to be a more fruitful opportunity—for the company and for me.

I felt like I was running a race. At the starting line, engine revving (adrenaline, that is) and ready to hit the ground running. Oh, I did that all right. I hit the pavement scouting out potential advertisers. But I didn't realize how difficult it is to sell air. Compared to my first sales job, this one was tough. There were no existing files to build from. No calling lists. Just a big, fat phone book that was plopped on our desks after two days of training (a.k.a. boot camp for selling airtime.) And it didn't even have a pretty bow tied on top of it (I'm one for presentation; obviously, they weren't).

If I had had some money and extra time I could have taught management a course in presentation, but I decided to save my breath and, instead, poured it into the phone book. I would literally flop it open to a page, close my eyes and "let my fingers do the walking" Ouija-board style. After opening my eyes, I looked at the business I selected and dialed the phone number before talking myself out of it.

Although I made a very minimal amount of sales during my four months at the radio station, I'm proud to say hardly anyone hung up on me. I actually had some pretty pleasant conversations with business owners (everyone always enjoys talking about themselves). Some people were so enthusiastic and interesting I found myself going to their business and buying a few things from them.

After four months of barely meeting my sales quota, I was gently given a goodbye (a.k.a. you're fired). I was inwardly thrilled. Yes, the umbilical cord of selling airtime was cut from me. Now I could do what I really wanted to do—nothing! I wanted to be free. To enjoy the sunshine, eat my lunch at a park, walk my dog, take afternoon naps and have absolutely no obligations. And that was exactly what I got.

I remember walking out of the radio office building with a huge grin on my face. I felt light, elated and *free*. Thank you, God! It called for an ice cream run, followed by a trip to the park where I sat in my car, enjoying my mint chocolate chip ice cream and the silence.

One drawback I had quickly learned by selling radio ads was how repelled I was at listening to the radio—any station. They *all* caused me stress and this is so not the purpose of listening to the radio—okay, heavy metal would cause me stress—but certainly jazz and classical stations shouldn't. I just enjoyed the silence and looked through my windshield that needed to have a few smashed bugs removed and reminded myself to take a trip to a carwash.

I truly felt content, like everything was okay. No stress. I hadn't felt that free and happy since the summer before my senior year at NMSU. Funny how I look back at that particular summer as a milestone, a mile marker to base my future endeavors on. It was a great summer and I was grateful to be experiencing a moment in my life that was reminding me of it. In some ways, I could freeze-frame this particular moment, I thought, but, somehow, I think my ice cream cone would not concur. Ironic thoughts—freezing time but ice cream melts.

While I was sitting in my car under a huge shade tree, praying a bird wouldn't use my car as a target, I thought it would be nice to bring my dog, Tigger, for a walk here in the evening. And we did just that.

TIGGER

"Expect your every need to be met, expect the answer to every problem, expect abundance on every level, expect to grow spiritually."

—Eileen Caddy

I never realized how vital a role a dog could play in a relationship, probably because Tigger was my first dog. I got him when I bought my house at the age of 24. He definitely was the best part of living in my home.

It was also the loneliest time of my life. After I got rid of my boyfriend, Josh, the house felt so empty. I thought Josh and I were on our way to getting married. We'd been together for three years and, my gosh, wasn't owning a house a move in the right direction to marriage? I'm not sure if I read that concept in a book or if I had created the idea in my mind. Either way, after three years, Josh was out of the picture.

Being single at age 24 was something I was definitely not prepared for. The friends I had from my prior job had disappeared. I honestly thought that everyone in their twenties had either moved away or were hiding under rocks because I couldn't find *anyone* in my age range to hang out with—a frustrating and lonely experience. Those two words became my best friends over the next several years and my new, decorative motif became snotty tissues haphazardly thrown all over the floor.

If dogs could talk, I wonder what Tigger would have said during that time. He looked so wise, like Yoda, and I was so pitiful.

"Tigger, I don't know what to do," I said to him as I cupped his cute face in my hands and stared into his brown eyes. With tears pouring down my face, I explained to Tigger what had happened with Josh and why he wasn't in our life anymore.

An inspiration struck me. I found several photos I'd taken of Josh.

"Okay Tigger," I said, "Let out your aggression. I give you full permission to pee all over these photos. Oh wait! Let me put down some newspaper first. I don't want to mess up the wood floors."

Tigger looked at me. I looked at him. "Well, you first," I said. "You have better aim. Now's your chance for paybacks. He didn't just hurt me when he left. He hurt us. And we're a team. So pee away."

He sniffed the stack of photos and puts his paw on one photo in particular and licked it, as if to kiss it.

"No, no," I said. "Piss, not kiss!"

I took a closer look at the photo. It was taken during my senior year at college. We'd been dating about a year and we looked so happy, so *right* together. My hands shook. All that was left from that memory was this photo? A future in the making and all I have to show for it is this photo? I was in shock.

It wasn't supposed to be this way, I thought. God, why did you let this happen? What did I do that was so bad that I'm being punished by being left alone?

You're never alone, Michelle, a voice said. All you

have to do is reach out and start talking. I'm here with you now during your pain and I'll be here for you, always. I love you and I will not abandon you. There are things you may not understand now, but just remember this—everything happens for a reason. People are in our lives for a reason, a season or a lifetime. Josh was in your life for a reason.

I was startled. "Oh."

Looking around, I slowly turned my head to look at Tigger. He raised an ear. "Honey, did you just hear what I heard?"

He was unresponsive, so I gather he didn't.

All righty then, I thought. I am officially losing it. I'm hearing voices in my head and this is not good. It must be the stress. Oh, dear Lord, please don't let it be some satanic cult thing taking over my brain.

I hurriedly packed up the photos of Josh and me, and I took a trip down memory lane to the trash can and dumped them all in one big crashing cymbal sound and slammed down the lid—tight. That voice can stay in there, as well. I'm done with Josh.

Back in the house, I let out a loud sigh. I rolled my head side-to-side and the tension in my shoulders released.

"This was a good thing," I said to Tigger. "Moving forward. Clearing out the old to make room for the new. Go us! Right, Tigger. High ten."

10:00 PM arrived. Yawning, I decided to call it a night. I'd start fresh in the morning by clearing out the remainder of Josh's lurking memory. Getting rid of the photos wasn't so bad, I thought, although some of the frames were really nice. Damn! I should've kept those, at least.

"No, Michelle, let it go," my voice said. "If you're going to get rid of Josh, you've got to get rid of all of him—frames and all. There'll be more photos down the road."

23

With that thought I brushed my teeth and headed to bed.

•••

It was Saturday morning. I went over the day's plans with Tigger. I was going to clean out the house and get rid of anything that was a reminder of Josh. Fortunately, it's a small house, I thought. It would go quickly. Wrong.

I can't believe how many things I still have that he gave me, I thought. It's like a museum, with photos scattered along shelves and the books he gave me and stacks of Hallmark cards from every holiday and those "I'm sorry" and "just because" occasions. I'm a fool for sentimental things, I admitted.

"I know, I know. It's just paper. Get rid of it," I said to Tigger and for the air to hear.

Around me, I made a semi-circle stack of Josh memorabilia. Three years, I reminisced. My longest relationship with a guy so far. Well, at least I can be thankful that we didn't have kids.

"Tigger," I said, "You are my child. And I'm so very thankful you're in my life."

Being motivated to do things has always been a positive aspect of my personality. Once I'm focused on doing something—watch out. But cleaning up the mess from my past was different. It proved to be my most difficult task yet, and it took a monumental force to get my butt up off the floor and grab some trash bags. I felt like I was tied to a heavy weight, wanting to drown myself in Josh's memories displayed on the den floor. It felt like he'd died. Only it wasn't physical, it was an emotional death. And I couldn't let go.

I sobbed and sobbed and made another display of tissue snot art all over the floor. "Nobody's here to help me," I angrily cried out into a tissue. "I can't do this alone. I don't have the strength. Please, someone help me."

The voice returned. "I'm here, Michelle. I'm always here. Just like I told you last night."

"Then why am I left alone to clean up the mess from Josh and my relationship?"

"Some things, no matter how painful they are at first are the most healing things. Take as much time as you need. Take care of yourself."

I stood up, picked up the wads of soppy tissues and dumped them in the trash. I grabbed a trash bag in the kitchen and like a whirlwind, I threw everything that surrounded me on the floor into the bag—and I didn't look twice.

My inner conversations had given me an unknown inner strength to take the next step in my cleaning-up process. And as on the previous night, I made another trip to the trashcan, lifted the lid and chucked the bag inside, not looking back. I slammed the lid down and made my way back inside with a lighter bounce in my step. An unbearable weight had been lifted from my body. It was almost like I had been carrying another body around—Josh's. Damn, it felt good to be released of that.

SCHOOL DAYS

"Never look back unless you are planning to go that way."
                                    —Henry D. Thoreau

While I sat on the den floor in my home, my mind began to wander to my past—back to when I was totally happy, carefree and had no bills. Just one endless summer at New Mexico State University in Las Cruces, New Mexico, and 110-degree daily temperatures to contend with.

That was the ultimate summer of summers. I had friends to hang out with until late in the night, talking and laughing. I thought it would never end.

It's what I imagine when certain songs come on the radio and take me back to that summer of 1995. I had two classes per five-week summer school session and tons of time for fun. As the saying goes, "You never know what you've got till it's gone." This is so true.

My eyes moistened with fresh tears and I could feel a smile appear on my face. I miss that summer at NMSU, I thought. And there's no going back. There were only memories to envelop my mind. I wiped my right cheek with the back of my hand.

Out of four years in college, I got to experience only

one good summer—the one I still reminisce about. That's it, I thought. I felt gypped. I never got to experience the full college experience—the *fun* part—and I went to a *party* school. How in the world did I manage to avoid the social side?

Graduating with honors was great, but if I could go back, I wouldn't have isolated myself to get A's. But what about the fun? And friends? That's a void I'll forever have in my life. Ironic, eh? Some wish they'd dedicated themselves more to getting good grades. I wish I'd learned how to relax, have fun, and meet people and laugh.

I also remember when I first arrived at NMSU. Against suggestions from other people, my roommate was my best friend from high school. It was great for a couple of months until we started having disagreements. I knew I had to make a change. The tension when we were around each other got unbearable and I felt anxious. We never fought like this in high school—then again, we didn't live together in high school!

I decided to go through sorority rush and pledged Alpha Chi Omega. The class load hadn't hit me yet, so I had plenty of time to socialize and relax. If this is college life, I thought, then—hello—am I ever glad to be here. This is a piece of cake. It was the first time in my life when I felt completely free. No one was telling me what to do, I was just free to be and explore and grow. No bills, no stress and cute cowboys *everywhere.* Everything was new and fresh: people, classes, everything was interesting. I felt so alive!

I had my first encounter with a cowboy when I joined the sorority. My best friend and I went to a dance on campus (we had made amends), and every time I hear a Garth Brooks or George Strait song I still think of that dance and meeting Joe, my cute cowboy.

Joe was a perfect gentleman and patient as he taught me

how to two-step, waltz and cotton-eye Joe. It felt so right being in his arms, and we went to several parties together. He even brought me coffee when I was studying. He was a great first boyfriend for me in college. I'll never forget him. He made me feel special—like a lady. I thought *all* guys I met after him would treat me the same way.

I didn't realize until after I graduated from college that Joe was raised the right way, and I was a fool for letting him go. I thought my studies were much more important than dating someone. He was the kindest, most thoughtful young man I had met at NMSU. And boy, could he country dance.

For the two months we dated he definitely made an impression on me. I wish all the men I had dated while I was in college would have been required to go through a "gentleman's school" in the little town Joe was from. He was just interested in getting to know me as a person, and I never felt he was taking advantage of me—one of the nicest feelings in the world.

That feeling of love and freedom didn't reenter my life until my senior year at NMSU. No work then, just a light load of three classes and looking for a job after graduation. I was determined I was going to be successful, make my mark in the corporate world, and make my friends and parents proud.

It was a fast, fun year with new changes on the horizon and I was ready to hit the ground running in Corporate America. Between reading textbooks, writing term papers and stressing about getting employed (somewhere prestigious, of course), I was more than ready to earn some money.

Funny thing, no one had told me there's a price to pay for working in Corporate America. That you sell your soul and they work you like a dog, seeing how far they can stretch you until you break.

I was naïve. I thought my first job was going to be similar to my parents' work environment, where people were happy to see me and I felt relaxed and welcomed. Why would things change for me when I started working? I couldn't wait to earn a paycheck.

My boyfriend, Josh, and I had been dating my entire senior year. I was nervous about confronting him about the future of our relationship. I didn't know if I could handle us breaking up, but it was inevitable the conversation would have to occur—the sooner, the better. So, before spring break I let him know what my plans were. I had applied to at least a dozen different advertising jobs. And I wasn't particular where I would end up living. I just knew I wanted Josh to be by my side.

Josh said wherever I ended up would be fine. He was planning to enroll in college, so he applied at the universities where I was hoping to find employment. I couldn't believe how accommodating he was.

This is what love is about, I thought. Making compromises. I'd never experienced true love before. I was really lucky to find such a great, understanding guy as Josh. I just knew we were going to have a great future together.

MEN

"Do what you can with what you have where you are."
—Theodore Roosevelt

"Josh, I'm lonely," I said. "Why don't we ever spend time together anymore? You know, go out and do things—eat and have fun. I miss that. I miss that about us, Josh. You're always having to work weekends. And as predictable as any other Friday night—I'm in the damn laundry room listening to the churning of our clothes and on guard so no one takes off with them. This really sucks. Our relationship once was filled with laughter and fun at college. I really miss that. Why did it have to change?"

I didn't think *I'd* changed that much. It must be him, I thought. If this is our future together—loyal woman that I am—then I'm in for a lifetime of loneliness, sadness and frustration.

There was no out for me. Once I was committed to something or someone I stuck to them like fly paper. I don't know where I learned this, but unfortunately I hadn't learned the difference between quitting and moving on with my life.

I was determined to make our relationship work no

31

matter how many Oprah shows and Dr. Phil books it took. I thought my relationship was my thing to fix.

"Look Josh," I said. I was excited and hopeful that he'd be game to hear what I had to share. "Dr. Phil encourages open, honest communication with your partner. This is definitely what we're lacking."

Josh rolled his eyes. "Michelle," he said in a bored tone, "our relationship is fine. Everyone goes through tough times. We'll get through this. And we sure don't need some book telling us how to fix our relationship."

I felt deflated. My attempt to bring hope back into our relationship left me feeling like a sad child. I tried, I thought. Why didn't he like my idea? Where did our team effort go?

I didn't share our relationship problems with anyone. I thought, like work, everyone had problems and it was just part of being in a committed relationship. Yeah, committed for life. My jail sentence.

Josh was only half-listening as he undid his tie and kicked off his shoes after a six-hour shift selling shoes at a local department store.

The sales side of me emerged as I continued to read from Dr. Phil's book. "We can do this, Josh. We just need to make more time for us to go out and do things." "That's a nice thought, Michelle," Josh said, "but between school and work, I'm exhausted."

"Well, maybe you could cut back on your work hours. Don't you think our relationship is worth it?"

Silence.

"Josh?" I closed the book on my lap and looked at the title. My tears splashed on the front cover, blurring the words and the image of Dr. Phil. Was there something I wasn't seeing clearly? Something I wasn't understanding? This was the longest relationship I'd been in—three years. I thought for sure we were destined to get married.

Like a dead weight, I trudged to our bedroom and plopped myself on the fluffy southwest-style comforter. "I don't understand. Why is everything such a struggle?"

I sobbed into the comforter so it would muffle my voice as I buried my face in the comforter to let the tears soak up the pain. Work. Josh. My parents. I felt like I was pushing a boulder up a mountain barefoot with the sun beating down on me. There's no one behind me to encourage me along, I thought.

After a while, Josh came into the bedroom. After sitting next to me he rubbed my back like a mother soothing an upset baby. "Michelle," he said, "I didn't mean to upset you, but lately you get so over emotional about things that we talk about. I feel I never say the right thing and you end up crying.

"It's hard for me to share things with you because I never know what kind of response I'll get. I feel like I'm playing dodge ball, hoping to say the right thing to avoid being bombarded by your intense, uncontrollable emotions.

"I don't remember our relationship being this difficult last year when you were in college, Michelle. But things have definitely changed. I'm here for the long haul."

"Long haul? What the hell is *that* supposed to mean?" I turned onto my back and propped myself on my elbow. "Long haul? Well, isn't that romantic?" I said sarcastically—a skill I developed over the years to protect my true feelings.

I knew Dr. Phil would not approve of my behavior, but I didn't care. An immediate thought of smacking the book hard in Josh's face entered my mind. Instead I threw the damn book at him. Maybe he'd get some ideas on compassion and understanding me after reading a few chapters, I thought. Insensitive jerk, I said to myself.

I felt so weak from crying. "Just get out of here. Leave me alone." I wanted to give up. My body was limp, like overcooked spaghetti. Finally, exhausted from crying, I drifted off to sleep, alone.

I ruminated. Why was I in this relationship? Company was the answer. Plain and simple. I didn't want to live alone. I was an only child, so living independently was no problem, but coming home to an empty place didn't sit right with me. I should have gotten a dog. I was chicken. I was scared. I didn't know what to do with my time.

I had racing and nerve-wracking thoughts about work that regularly drove me into extreme states of paranoia and anxiety, which no one saw, except Josh. He was there for me through all my crying and anger spells, my wanting to give up, my not understanding the real world, and my regular conflicts with co-workers. It was all too much for me to handle.

I considered Josh to be my protective blanket—there to shelter me from the pain and to listen while I sobbed for hours. He would hold me close, making me feel that nothing or no one could harm me. But he never understood why I got upset so regularly. Nor did I.

The stress from work and my co-workers, our apartment living environment and chores set me off on a daily emotional high-and-low roller coaster ride. Neither of us knew when my emotions would strike or which emotion would take center stage. I thought it was how my personality was forming and that I better get used to it.

Interestingly, thoughts of visiting my doctor never entered my mind. I looked fine on the outside, so how could I justify seeing my doctor for unseen symptoms? In my world, my behavior was normal. Everyone had ups and downs. The only difference was that I had highs and lows. It was like comparing an eczema rash to a third-degree burn.

MEN

Everything was a trigger that sent my mood spiraling—downward to depression during the fall and winter months—literally September 1 through February 28—and then upward to a hypo-manic state from March 1 to August 31.

Looking back, those highs and lows were more regular and predictable with the alternating seasons when I was in college. I thought the lack of daylight in the fall and winter caused me to have Seasonal Affective Disorder (SAD), which explained why I was irritable and reclusive, craved sweets and carbohydrates, and felt lethargic for six months out of the year. I was paranoiac and thought my classmates were talking about me.

But I poured all my energy into my books, which—ironically—is probably the reason I graduated with honors. When spring arrived and daylight hours increased, the symptoms cast aside their dark shadow and I felt like me again. I was sociable, had more energy and creativity, and I slept and ate less. School demands didn't cause me as much stress. My paranoia disappeared. I felt great!

●●●

God, I hate this room, I thought, with its ugly, greenish-yellow paint and six washing machines and three dryers. My Friday night entertainment is absolutely and utterly pathetic. I hate feeling trapped in this ugly jail cell while Josh has his freedom of going to work.

My disappointment and anger encompassed me as I threw the whites, darks and towels into their appropriate washing machines. This is it, I thought. Is this what our relationship has come to? I fought hard not to have tears of anger break through my tear-stained face as I added laundry soap and fabric softener to each machine. I'm 22 years old. I should be out with friends, laughing, dancing and having fun. I should let Josh do his own laundry. Let him go naked, for all I care.

For two years, Friday nights were the loneliest, most predictable days of the week. After laundry time, I'd sink myself into a God-awful, brown recliner—a "gift" from Josh's mother—that didn't quite fit our décor.

Yeah, right, I thought. This chair hasn't moved in two years. I fear it will either disintegrate from mold or unsightly critters will come out of it. What kind of mother would dump such crap on her son? Guess there were still some things I had yet to learn about Josh.

"Thanks, Mom," he had said.

Thanks, Mom? For this piece of shit furniture? Are you kidding me? "You're not actually going to bring that thing into our apartment, are you?" I had said.

"Oh, Michelle," he had said. "Relax. It was a gift."

"Well, don't bother bringing it upstairs, the dumpster's much closer. It's the bin next to the laundry room. Yes, that's right. The room where I live one night a week. Maybe you can put the damn chair in there so I can wallow in comfort in your mom's 'gift' while I listen to the churning laundry machine." Could my life suck any more?

My early encounters with the washing machines were tolerable. Although it wasn't on my fun list, it was something that I did in college. I was proud that I could last three weeks before having to visit the Laundromat on campus, five minutes from my student apartment. It was clean and several machines were available at the same time. I was able to leave my clothes while doing other things, like visiting friends or watching TV.

I must admit, I was a bit spoiled by my mom. She'd do my laundry for me when I was growing up, when I came home from college, and when I returned to living at home. I definitely appreciated it because I grew to really dislike doing laundry, which put a sour taste in my mouth and reminded me of my horror days at the "Sad Café."

How I longed for those days with my mom. I had never fully appreciated her for the time, energy and love she put into making sure I had clean clothes—a task that was so simple, yet said so much.

My throat burned as I tried to hold back the beginning stage of tears. "I can't keep doing this laundry work." I said, sobbing with my head on the washing machine. "It's too much."

Anger, frustration and loneliness boiled up inside me. Round and round the tears welled up and new emotions surfaced. When will I run out of tears? I've never cried so much in my life, I thought. The internal pain is killing me. And nobody sees it. Nobody cares. Everyone has their own problems to deal with. I've just got to pull myself together and deal with this the best way I can.

Like someone hiding an alcohol problem, I hid my tears from everyone—only there was no twelve-step program for chronic criers.

I was running on auto-pilot, and it was not glamorous. I was a walking zombie. Dead on the inside and stressed out on the outside, I didn't care about anything anymore. I was in survival mode. I had no one to talk to about the feelings I was having. Don't all working people feel this way? I thought. I believed everyone was as stressed and unhappy as I was. But that gave me no comfort, only a sense of wanting to retreat back to my college days.

If I would have allowed God to have a presence during this stage of my life, I believe He would have shared a bit of knowledge with me: "The pressure on you may be intense. A half-dozen joy stealers may be waiting outside your door, ready to pounce at the first opportunity. However, nothing can rob you of your hold on grace, your claim to peace, or your confidence in God without your permission. Choose joy. Never release your grip."

...

On the way home from work every Friday night I would buy groceries, finding whatever was on sale in the weekly ads—our menu for the week. I had no mental or physical energy to exert in cooking anything beyond simple meals, such as sloppy Joes, spaghetti, burritos. Just get me home was my motto.

After collapsing into a dining room chair, I stared at the empty chair where Josh would sit. Sometimes he came home for dinner, but more frequently he didn't. I'd heat up a microwave meal, letting the tears trickle down my cheeks onto my napkin while I stared at my pathetic dinner. I never ate like this before. I'm so alone, I thought. I have no one to turn to for friendship, for anything. Even my landlord doesn't like me. How can I keep going on like this? I have no control over anything in my life. And for *this* I went to college and graduated with honors?

Honestly, I thought, I just want one night a week when I can go out with friends. Okay, this sounds like a great idea, but where do I find friends? My college friends are gone, in other states, with their new post-grad lives. I have no one. No one person, that is. But I have TV. My friend. My comforter. My pacifier that drowns out the noise in my brain—my fears and anger. Just let the TV mesmerize you and smooth everything over and relax. And I did, until each Monday morning.

Looking back, how I did what I did—work in advertising for five years— I'll never know. A miracle comes to mind. At work I had crying spells, and my anxiety fed off my paranoia. I thought my co-workers were conspiring to get me fired. Upon returning home after work every day, I was physically and emotionally drained, my brain flooded with negative thoughts. I was a mess—an emotionally unstable, miserable, lonely mess.

It still amazes me how I lasted as long as I did working in advertising. Five words were the key: monthly rent or mortgage payment.

I really enjoyed my work. My clients were great, and I was like a daughter to many of them. I enjoyed getting to know them and their businesses. Collecting their monthly invoices was secondary to my visits. Unfortunately, I didn't quite feel the same love back at the office, or was it "hell hole?" As I said, "I love my clients, but my boss is a B*&#$%." Truth hurts, I thought. Ouch!

"Just another manic Monday" by Cindy Lauper was my theme song. Her plea became mine, and I wondered, why can't *my* life be like a never-ending Sunday? If I lived on my own planet it would be possible. But until I figure out a way to get the hell outta this job, it's off to work.

6:00 AM Monday.

My body was bone tired and sore from a night of tossing and turning. I was unable to fully relax and I unknowingly contracted my muscles throughout the night. It was hard to walk. I felt like I had arthritis. I'm 23, I thought. This is all in my head. I looked at myself in the bathroom mirror. I really looked at the reflection of my hazel eyes. They're sad and frustrated, but mostly sad. I never really stared at my reflection before, I thought. Well, when I pop a zit I do, but never to analyze my eye expression.

Freshly brewed tears made trail marks down my face. I felt numb. And sore. And trapped. *This* is why I went to college? *This* is why I studied so hard? To graduate with honors and now to be treated like shit by my co-workers? I want to go back, I thought. "I can't do this anymore." I cried at my reflection in the mirror.

Sobbing, I sat on the toilet seat with my hands cupping my eyes. "I don't understand," I said. "I just want out. But I can't. I'm stuck. I have rent to pay and other bill responsibilities. I just--"

More uncontrollable, wracking sobs came up from deep inside me. I didn't care if my boyfriend could hear through the closed bathroom door. "I have no one to turn to. No one to fix things. It's over. This is the rest of my life. And I'm only 23."

It was sadness like I'd never experienced before. Sadness I didn't share with anyone. Not even God. Oh, He knew my pain, but I never reached out for His help. It never occurred to me to pray—probably because of all the noise in my brain. It never fully rested and neither did the rest of me. I always felt "on." I was constantly thinking, rethinking, reliving and fearing the future. Basically, I ruminated about any thought from my past or in the future. There was no living in the present for me.

I couldn't remember a time that I was completely in the present moment—to just be, to live as a "human being" and not as a "human doing." I was a robot dictated to by co-workers and my uncontrollable thoughts. They told me what to do, when and how to act. It was pathetic. But I did it anyway. I so completely lost myself in others' wishes that I literally turned over my existence to them, allowing them to mold me into whatever they thought would be acceptable to them. Honestly, I just gave up. It was easier that way. I felt so dead inside, why should it matter how my outside appeared?

...

MEN

Control. The word brought excitement to my mind. I'd done control a million times since I was 11-years old. Although it was in remission, my anorexia eating disorder could return as easily as picking up the phone—just the "high" I needed to let me escape all the negativity and lack of control that was happening to me.

Oh, they–including Josh, co-workers, parents and society—may be able to dictate every other area of my life, I thought, but how much I eat, they can't touch. No one can force me to eat. It's mine. All mine.

No one knew for a few months. No one was around to see my unhealthy eating patterns. I felt happy. Elated. Watching the number on my bathroom scale go lower and lower each week brought me joy. Then I went to weighing myself every day. If the number on my scale met my expectation, then all was well in my world.

Now, this is living, I thought. I look great. Josh is surely going to notice and want to be seen with me in public. My weight loss will surely bring us closer together intimately. Weight loss was the answer to my prayers. I wasn't overweight to begin with, so achieving the magic number of 127 pounds was pure joy for my eyes. That goal, like a present waiting to be revealed, was what got me out of bed each morning.

Josh had no idea what was going on. I hid the scale under the bathroom sink counter under some towels. My parents never said anything. Neither did my co-workers.

It was my secret that no one knew about. One that almost killed me.

A WALK IN THE PARK

"I have made my world and it is a much better world than I ever saw outside."

—Louise Nevelson

Ding, ding. "Ice cream, anyone?" The sound of the ice cream truck with its familiar summer sound circling the park reminded me of happy childhood times. I felt a big Popsicle grin on my face. Sunlight hit my face, warming me. I resonated from the inside out. With Tigger leading the way around the park it was easy to get wrapped up in the present moment and to just "be."

Whatever work problem, relationship problem or money problem, everything faded away except the present. When *was* the last time I had experienced this feeling? I didn't recall. But I absolutely loved it—the freedom, the peace of mind, the happy, carefree signs of spring surrounded me. And all was well in my world.

Tigger and I had been going to the park for a couple of months and we had seen many familiar faces. People played on volleyball leagues, small children played with glee on the jungle gym, and yes, lots of dog walkers strolled around the park that drew them from all over the neighborhood. Tigger enjoyed his daily encounters with the small dogs, especially a couple of cute, small females. And he let the big dogs know who was in charge by growling and lunging at them. I think he was even successful in scaring off a few.

Tigger, my super-protector and best friend, loved that park where people were so friendly. While I was chatting with the regulars, Tigger left messages on trees near the walk path and he got to know the other dogs well or just patiently sat and waited for me to finish my conversation.

Day after day, Tigger and I had our walk date at the park. People of various ages were attracted to this park for different reasons such as sports and—could it be—to meet new friends? Honestly, I thought, if Tigger could do it, why not me? Of course, Tigger being a natural leader, would take a beeline towards a cute girl dog with an equally cute guy owner.

I met many men that way, but the most interesting and memorable man was Warren, an older man about 55 years old—old enough to be my father. We met one day when Tigger pulled me towards him. He had two large dogs and I was sure Tigger would kindly introduce himself by barking and lunging at them. He just sniffed them. Amazing.

Warren was kind and a good listener. I enjoyed the company. Day after day we had our daily talk and walk sessions. I began to think of him as a school-of-life teacher. He spoke from his heart and appreciated my sense of humor and insight. Almost from the beginning we felt comfortable in each other's presence.

After knowing him for a month I invited him over for a barbeque, and he agreed. I had invited a few neighbors over and we enjoyed each other's company. And yes, dogs were invited. It was a pleasant Sunday afternoon. After a few hours the neighbors left and Warren stayed to help me clean up.

It was the first time he'd been to my house. He washed the dishes, and I dried and put them away. I had a small kitchen—cozy for two people. We talked and laughed and I felt completely relaxed. I can't tell you how rare it is for me to talk to a man, have it start as a friendship and stay as a friendship. And I didn't pick up on vibes from Warren indicating otherwise.

When we finished the dishes, we moved to the living room to collapse. The afternoon had zapped us both of energy. I thought I would definitely sleep well that night.

•••

As the days of spring graced into summer, April came and left with a light breeze and summer bloomed in full color. Warren and I continued our walks together. Tigger adored him because Warren often brought treats for Tigger, which was really sweet and won my heart. If a way to a man's heart is through his stomach, then a way to a woman's heart is through how her dog is treated.

He never asked about my employment, marital status or financial status. He definitely was not caught up in the rat race—a breath of fresh air. I felt I could share *anything* with him and he would accept and encourage me and let me be me. The relationship was very liberating, and I felt myself becoming more creative with my emotional shadow coat being lifted off me.

Warren was the first man in a long time, perhaps ever, to accept me as I was. Releasing my emotions, although leaving me feeling exposed, didn't scare or bother me. Should I bury them? Burn them? Release them? Yes, release them, I thought. It was an inner freeing feeling. It was easier to breathe.

45

...

It amazes me to this very day how quickly some friendships are formed. As if joined by the hip, I couldn't tell where I began and Warren ended. Our communication was wonderful. Every time I saw him I craved to learn more about him because he was very much interested in hearing more about *my* life.

I was growing quite fond of him, but not in a romantic way—more of a comfy couch sort of way—something that's always there when you need it (especially when you're tired and can't stay on your feet any longer) and something that supports you and conforms to your needs. Yes, Warren was quickly becoming my human couch (although I didn't divulge this for fear he'd get pissed off and call me a lamp, or worse—a dining room table). I've never been referred to as a piece of furniture, but nonetheless, I kept that thought to myself.

Driving home from the park each day with Tigger, I was greeted by a beautiful home, but one that was absorbed by loneliness. In my home, several things that I owned were beautiful but, unfortunately, talking to furniture only goes so far. The closest I came to communicating with technology was whenever AOL greeted me with "You've Got Mail."

How easy it was to become addicted to that voice and everything it had to offer. Pick your poison: E-bay or endless dating services. Tempting? You bet. I could feel my body becoming drained while I spent almost every night cruising the net, looking to fill the void in my life. I think of all those beautiful summer nights that I spent glued to my computer monitor for some sort of answer to pop up on the screen. Answer to what? I asked. I don't know, I answered.

But reflecting about the park and how I felt around Warren is what kept me awake many nights, reviewing our conversations in my head and thinking about what I wanted to share with him the next day. I felt alive—like a child who's just met her first best friend.

In addition to the countless nights I was unable to sleep, I was amazed how I could bounce out of bed the next morning feeling refreshed and ready to rock and roll. I was neither hungry nor tired. Having so much time on my hands—since eating and sleeping were out of the picture—I began creating things, many of which I couldn't wait to share with Warren.

At the park, I shared with him a few of my ideas over a period of several weeks. He listened attentively and although he didn't say much, I didn't pick up on the worrisome look on his face that emanated "Danger, we're going down!" He didn't want to squash my ideas for fear of sabotaging our friendship.

He listened with each passing day as more ideas poured out from my mouth. It was dizzying, even for me, to keep up. Warren very much wanted to help me, but he didn't want to tell me that I wasn't well and that I'd better check myself into the nearest mental health hospital. He was right. That definitely would not have been well received by me.

Every day that Warren saw me at the park brought him a sense of relief. A big sigh...and off we went again. Only then, along with the endless creative projects, came rapid talking (talking as fast as I was thinking) and hallucinating.

•••

Reliving this experience in my mind is one thing, but to put it on down on paper to share with everyone is rather embarrassing. I ask you, the reader, to please keep in mind while reading this portion that I was definitely NOT in my right mind. I was physically there, but my mind was not.

"It's a date" quickly escalated to "time to move in" and cohabitate as long as possible (his decision). His reasoning? Beats the hell out of me. He knew something was wrong with me, and he was going to use it to his advantage.

He told no one and I thought I was fine. He was around my house quite a bit, which actually was a good thing. He made sure I ate—cooking meals on my stove and making sure I didn't physically harm myself (although, I don't recall this thought even entering my mind).

The first day he moved in he brought his toothbrush. Thoughtful, since I don't share mine with anyone. I guess he knew. Yep. He was a light traveler, all right. (He lived only two miles from my house, so everything was nearby for him).

He stayed with me for five days and four nights. Oh, boy. The nights—okay, please read this with an open mind and try not to get too grossed out. One of the symptoms of being in a manic state is an increased libido, or sex drive. Fortunately, being 55-years old had left him sterile (thank you, God) because for the first time in my life, I wasn't using any form of birth control. My biggest concern was getting pregnant. I let him know that and he said it wasn't a problem—the *only* truth he told me and I'm grateful for that.

As if I was trying to seduce Warren, I bought scented candles and put them on my jewelry box on my bedroom dresser. The wax melted all over the top of my jewelry box. I didn't even bother to blow out the candles. I could've burned my house down. I wore a turquoise negligee I thought would enhance the mood. Yep. It did that all right. He almost crushed me, his weight was easily double mine. Help! Air! I need air!

Throughout the next five days and four nights I quickly fell in love with Warren. Our age difference didn't matter. He knew me like no other man had and I was convinced that God had brought us together. The infatuation rapidly grew to a reality in my mind. I was absolutely elated and I told him on day four that I was in love with him and we were getting married. I whipped out a "to-do" list to prepare for the wedding. Oh, there were so many details to take care of—and I was just the person for the job.

I began with the obvious: "First off, I love you, honey, but the gut has got to go. You look like you're pregnant. Now, you can either have liposuction done, which would be faster, or join a gym. At any rate, I don't want you waddling down the aisle. If I'm gonna' look good, then you're gonna' look good.

"Okay, next. Get a haircut. And color your hair. Brown would be nice. It would match mine. We need to shave off some serious years here, Warren. I hope you're not taking any of this personally. You'll look so *trés* fabulous when I'm done with your makeover. And yes, the moustache has to go, as well.

"You should also check into getting some contacts. Those glasses really date you.

"I'll go ahead and make an appointment to get your teeth bleached. Don't worry, it's painless.

"And lastly, you'll need to go buy a tuxedo 'cause we're boardin' a plane to Hawaii tomorrow to get married."

"Chop chop. Rock n' roll here. Time is money and I gotta' go shopping for our honeymoon."

Warren looked at me like I'd flipped my lid. I suppose he took my suggestions as insults. Well, it would be an improvement, I thought. He just didn't realize it yet. Warren stomped out of the house all pissed off. I figured, oh shoot, this is what married people do. So we're just getting a head start.

I looked good. I just wanted *him* to look a little younger—not like he was my Grandpa—or Santa Claus. I didn't think I was asking for much. He was just being way too sensitive about the whole thing. I figured he went back to his house for the day and we'd talk later that evening.

• • •

So, off to Target to pick up a few items for our honeymoon. Time was of the essence so I double-parked in the fire zone, which I deemed was allowed for such emergencies. After leaving my car running with the front door open, I sprinted into the store with shopping list in hand and zeroed in on the shopping carts. Thus, I began my "mad woman shopping spree."

"Ma'am. You can't park your car out there in the fire zone," said the security guard who quickly caught up to me in the accessory department.

"Sure, I can," I said to the guard over my left shoulder. "I'll only be a few minutes. See, got my list here. I'll be out in a jiffy."

After grabbing a shopping cart and heading off to the first section of the store, my eyes were drawn towards the hats, bags, sunglasses, scarves and sandals—10 to 15 each. "Wow! This is fun!"

I got cart number one filled up. I thought I'd go grab cart number two and asked a customer as he was entering the store if he'd mind helping me with the cart. He just looked at me—and in a not very helpful way.

Oh, forget him, I thought. I need a team of shoppers to help me with the rest of the store. This is my honeymoon. It's going to be great! I just don't know how I'm going to

cover the entire store on my own. So little time. "Team—
need a team" kept racing through my mind while I was
stressing over what shopping still remained.

Three store managers showed up and asked me to leave
the store. I told them I couldn't. I wasn't done shopping. I
asked for their help, and they just looked at me—a little
scared—probably wondering what kind of drugs I was on.

It didn't take long for the Crisis Intervention Team
(CIT) to appear at my side. One minute I was trying on a
cute, floppy hat and sunglasses, and the next I was being
dragged out of Target by my arm like mothers do with their
children.

It hurt. I kept screaming, "You're squishing my muscles,
you're squishing my muscles!" Bad childhood memories
surfaced about my mom who used the same technique to
grab my attention in stores. Worked like a charm every
time. I wondered how the CIT guy knew about the same
technique. I was stripped of hat and sunglasses and was
less-than-graciously dragged out of Target.

I yelled, "Ow, damn. You're hurting me, you're hurting
me. You're not hearing me. Let me GO! Who the hell do
you think you are, anyway?

"I was in there minding my own business, doing some
shopping for my honeymoon, which—by the way—my fiancé and I are leaving tomorrow, and now you come along
and drag me out of the store. Who the hell are you? I hope
you've come to assist me with my shopping 'cause I've got
A LOT of territory to cover in there."

"Oh, silly me" I reasoned. I didn't realize the store
called for backup. "Thank you for coming," I said. "This
will work out great. The two of you CIT officers...by the
way, the uniform is a nice touch. That'll really get people's
attention and get them to move out of my way so my shopping can go faster. If you need some help with what to say,

let me know. I'm great with getting people's attention."

"Yes, we can see that, Michelle," the female officer replied.

"You know," I said. "I'm going to Hawaii tomorrow. My fiancé and I are getting married there. We're flying our entire guest list with us. They don't know this yet, though."

"Michelle, why don't you have a seat?" asked the same male CIT officer who had dragged me out by my arm. My car was still parked and waiting for me in the fire zone. How thoughtful of them to work with me here on my time-sensitive project. These people truly understand the urgency of my shopping trip. I'll have to keep this in mind for future vacations, I thought, smiling and with a sense of feeling important, like a movie star.

Looking back, he was a very kind man who didn't seem like a police type at all. But because I had never in my life come face-to-face with disobeying the law, I can't say I had any kind of reference to go by.

"You know, you're kinda cute," I told the officer. "You remind me of my R.A. at NMSU. He was very patient."

After listening to me ramble on about my wedding plans, my 55-year old fiancé and even inviting him to the wedding, I don't think anything I said surprised the officer by then.

A second officer had also been called for backup. She was a very nice woman, in her early thirties. She was very kind and patient, too. After asking my name, address and parents' names, phone number and address, she asked me to walk a straight line while touching my nose (I'd seen enough COPS shows to know she was checking whether I was drunk or on drugs.) I didn't need drugs—I was high as a kite on life. I'd never felt this giddy in my entire life. I loved it—nothing and no one could hurt me.

After the two officers conferred, the female officer decided she would take me to my parents' house. Before I got into the back seat of her police car she told me she needed to frisk me. With my hands on the passenger side of her car, she gently tapped the sides of my body. I could tell she felt uncomfortable, but I understood it was a matter of protocol. All she found was a tube of chapstick, which I got to keep with me.

It was late afternoon on the 23rd day of May 2001 when I got my first ride home in the backseat of a cop car. Oww! The plastic seat was hot, and the back of my legs were on fire. It could have been worse, though. At least I wasn't handcuffed. But the air conditioning didn't reach the back seat—that would be a perk of going to jail. I guess they didn't want to coddle would-be criminals with a free, air-conditioned ride to the county jail.

No air. Can't breathe. Melting, I thought.

It was only a 10-minute ride to my parents' house and the officer didn't even turn on the bubble gum lights. That was sort of a bummer. I wanted the whole pomp and circumstance.

"Come ON lady, can we speed it up, like TODAY?" I asked her to turn on the radio—country station, of course. I remember singing at the top of my lungs. I'm sure she was thankful for the glass barrier between us that muffled my off-key, blaring wannabe cowgirl voice.

Whether there was a radio in the car and whether it was even turned on, I don't know. But I was singing along to some great country songs that were whirling around my mind. Somehow I kept myself distracted enough to forget the sizzling sound of my body frying in the back seat.

I remember looking at the other cars and waving—smiling like I was a celebrity being chauffered to an event. First I waved like an excited child and then like Miss America. At stop lights, I stuck my tongue out at other cars.

Hey, this is fun! I thought. The officer had no idea what

I was doing, and even if she did, she didn't say anything. At one point, we passed a car and the people looked like mannequins. What in the world? I did a double take. That was weird, I thought.

We arrived at my parents' house around 5:30 PM. My dad was home from work. He was somewhat surprised (a huge understatement) to be greeted by a police officer, with me standing next to her. We went inside. I used the bathroom while they briefly discussed what had happened that afternoon. When I came out, the officer had left.

I told my dad the officer reminded me of my massage therapist—they looked similar. Too bad she'd already left. I wanted to schedule an appointment with her when we returned from our honeymoon. Oh well, I'm sure my dad had her phone number, I thought, and it'd be taken care of. How cool it was how everyone I was meeting had a double.

My dad sat down with me and tried to explain what I was experiencing was something that ran on his side of the family: bipolar disorder. He didn't know for sure if I had bipolar disorder, but he scheduled an appointment with my primary-care physician for the next morning.

Meanwhile, my mom and I were to meet at my house to go out to dinner. When I didn't appear, she drove to the restaurant, waited a half hour and then drove home crying, not knowing where I was. All the time, my dad and I were at home. When she arrived, I didn't understand why she was so upset.

"It's not every day that you get to ride in a cop car," I said.

Just about everything I said made my mom cry. I thought they were tears of joy–yeah, far from it. My dad managed to keep his composure, though, mainly because he'd seen this similar behavior before in his dad—my grandfather. And he knew if we could all hang in there until the next morning's appointment with my primary care physician, things would get better.

I couldn't sleep. I went to bed at 8:00 PM. At 10:00 PM I finally got up and watched the news with my parents. I didn't want to be alone, so I went into their bedroom and sat at the foot of their bed with a pillow propped up behind my head and their bedspread surrounding me like a cocoon. I felt protected by my parents and in my cocoon-like setup.

At 10:30 PM, my dad announced he was going to sleep. I kinda' freaked out. I didn't want to go back to my room alone with my racing thoughts. I couldn't relax. My brain was on overdrive and I didn't know how to relay that to him, so I went back to my room, scared, mad and disappointed. I felt like a young child again, being punished.

Like a puppy tucking its tail underneath I climbed back into bed and lay there, with my eyes wide open, staring at the ceiling and drumming my fingers on blankets I had pulled up to my chest. The drumming led to a song, which I couldn't get out of my head. I tossed. I turned. Damn this is annoying, I thought. Why won't my brain take a rest?

I got up, ate a bagel and turned on the television. I couldn't understand why I was eating breakfast at 2:00 AM. I was fascinated by the history channel (ironic, since I found my one college history course to be boring.)

And there I was writing as fast as I could. I was finding correlations between everything that was being said. I couldn't operate the VCR so, as fast as I could, I handwrote everything I heard. It would've been helpful to have a tape recorder, but I didn't want to wake my parents. I hoped I had enough pens and paper to make it through the night.

Sometime in the middle of the night, my parents came out to the living room to see what I was doing. I showed them my extensive notes on architecture in Roman times and the clothing styles. I thought I was Marilyn Monroe and needed protection from secret service agents so I wouldn't be recognized. I felt that every single fact on this program was being personally revealed to me.

I believe there are people here to help me along my journey. I'm becoming more aware of that and try to pay attention as to the information they share with me. What began the prior year as an occasional observation by the following May had progressed to a daily occurrence. Something that I craved. My connection to certain people kept me protected. Kept me alive. I trusted them with my life.

I believed there were two types of people–"straight talkers" and "go betweens." Straight talkers told me how it was. They were honest. People I trusted. Others were "go betweens." These were *definitely* the most interesting of conversations because they held "hidden meanings" for me to decode. These people were sent to me to deliver messages from God. Although I don't recall the conversations, I do remember thinking how very interesting they were.

My parents, Robert, Tigger and Warren were my "straight talkers." We had a secret pact. I remember asking Robert about "alive eyes" and "dead eyes." He knew *exactly* what I was talking about (this was before the serious hallucinations began.) "Alive eyes" had a sparkle in them, like Santa Claus. They lit up when people spoke. "Dead eyes" were zombie like, just an empty, flat stare.

As soon as I saw a "dead eyes" person, I diverted my eyes. These were devil people. They were here to consume me so I could no longer do my Godly work here on earth. My "go betweens" warned me of this. And they were everywhere. If I looked at them then I thought they'd change my eyes to "dead eyes" too. It was incredibly stressful. Who could I trust to look at? It was like playing dodge ball.

A WALK IN THE PARK

Actually, I was hallucinating both visually and auditorily. The TV was talking to me. I felt alive, alert and totally engrossed in the history program that was supposedly documenting my life. How much more could I ask for? I had just happened to flip to that channel only to discover that it was a documentary about my life. What are the chances of this happening? (Well, actually quite high if you're psychotic.)

My parents couldn't make any sense of the gibberish I'd written. I thought I was writing the most fascinating things and soon everyone would finally know about my secret life behind the scenes as Marilyn Monroe.

I finally fell asleep around 5:00 AM. At 8:00 AM, I was up again, exhausted and not thinking clearly at all. Not wanting to be recognized as Marilyn Monroe, I had packed disguise-clothes (shorts, t-shirt and sandals) so no one could determine my true identity.

It was all too soon. I had to protect myself. I felt it was going to be a challenge to explain to the world about how I had resurrected myself from the dead. I needed to remain as low-profile as possible. Having my parents escort me to keep me safe was a good plan.

My mom told me to get dressed because we were going to be leaving in a few minutes. I kept my nightgown on and put on my wedding shoes, sure that I would get my make-up and hair done before anything, so why bother getting dressed? When my parents saw me at the front door with my overnight bag in hand, my mom took me back to my room and told me to change into my shorts and t-shirt I had in my bag.

Okay, I thought. Whatever, people. I'm just trying to save us some time here. The hair and make-up people are waiting. This is just a waste of time.

I didn't even bother combing my hair or washing my

face. I guess you could say how I looked on the outside matched how I felt on the inside—shook up and wired, as if from drinking too much coffee.

Off we went to my first appointment to my make-up artist (in reality, my primary care physician.) As soon as the doctor arrived, I began telling her about my revelations from the prior night—being Marilyn Monroe in disguise, realizing I was God saving the world and curing all illnesses. No illnesses existed—I just wiped them off the slate. No more suffering. No more third-world countries starving for food and love, no divorces, no babies out of wedlock. No modern medicine necessary because there were no longer any illnesses.

As you may imagine, I was quite stressed by the huge responsibility I'd taken on. It was Jesus and me—disguised as Marilyn—working as a team that deemed it was time for our arrival on earth because of all the disarray and suffering. Of course, I had to take on a physical appearance, so people wouldn't be thinking they were hearing a voice and lose their minds. So Marilyn, it was!

I shared that information with my primary doctor. She immediately got on the phone and had me speak to another doctor. I felt my word was getting out, that people were whispering and pointing at me, saying, "Oh, my gosh. I can't believe it. God is actually here. And she's going to cure all illnesses."

The doctor couldn't stop watching me as I talked on the phone. I felt self-conscious, as if she were memorizing what I looked like. I remember telling her I liked her glasses. They were similar to mine.

The word began to spread like wildfire. I needed a team to help me spread the news to the masses. How? Who? My parents were my personal body guards, always protecting me. They led me wherever I needed to go, so I wouldn't have to think. Just move. And talk when needed. I was running on pure adrenaline, I couldn't stop talking. Ideas were spewing out of me, directly from my brain out my mouth. I was connecting the dots and seeing how the big picture of everything was coming together, like puzzle pieces floating down from the sky and snapping into place.

My "hair stylist" was a psychiatrist-in-training, I suppose. He asked a bunch of questions, many that duplicated those of doctor number one. I could tell he was fascinated by what I was telling him. He couldn't believe he was sitting in the same room as God.

I asked him if he wanted my autograph. He politely declined. Oh, well, his loss, I thought.

Like a game, the questions came fast, but I could shoot 'em down (answer them) as quickly as he asked them. What an adrenaline rush. I looked at my parents to make sure I was okay being where I was and that I was safe. One thing that drove my paranoia through the roof was that I was constantly afraid someone was going to kill me. I sat on edge, thinking my hair-stylist or psychiatrist was going to pull out a gun and shoot me. But, fortunately, my parents had given me a bullet-proof vest to wear prior to my appointment. Obviously, they had sensed something, too.

I told my mom, "Everything's going to be okay," and humbly added, "Who knew you'd given birth to God, huh?" This caused a whole other round of fresh tears. It was just too much for her to handle.

But I just said it to let her know that everything *was* going to be okay and with their help, we were going to make this world a better and more peaceful place to live. It was such an enormous task, but I knew I could do it. I just had to pace myself.

I was in full-blown mania (textbook case, the psychiatrist said). That meant: psychosis, rapid speech, no sleep, racing thoughts, numerous outlandish ideas, age of onset of 27, and being God. Interestingly, I read a couple of years later that people who are religious quite often take on a spiritual role, such as the Pope, Jesus, Mary, God or a disciple. And I thought I was the only God.

DIAGNOSIS

"Life is like an onion. You peel away one layer at a time
and sometimes you weep."

— Carl Sandburg

By 11 AM on May 24, 2001 we had been waiting in
the clinical psychologist's lobby for a while.
Eventually, the psychologist talked to me. After-
wards, my parents and I went home for lunch. I hardly ate
anything. I was really fidgety and restless. I had rapid
speech, spewing out ideas of whom to contact to help complete my mission, such as churches, schools and large areas
to hold meetings, including the Albuquerque Convention
Center and the UNM Pit—wherever large groups could be
gathered. I needed to move rapidly. Time was of the essence.
My mission was a domino effect that had to be implemented
as quickly as possible to spread the message around the
world.

But my parents said we had another appointment to go
to after lunch. I couldn't think of who we were to talk to
next.

While waiting for my appointment, my dad and I took a
short walk in our neighborhood with my dog, Tigger. While
my dad was walking him, I proceeded to raise people from

the dead by pointing at people's lawns and proclaiming, "There is no death or dying. No one suffers. You're not dead. Rejoice! I have come to save you. It's okay." I don't know if my dad was freaking out or if I was annoying him, but our brief walk was quite eventful and productive—for me, anyway.

After our walk, finally it was time to go to our next appointment. I demanded to know who wanted to meet with me. "People at the hospital." I started to freak out and back-pedaling saying "Oh, no we're not. I'm not going to any hospital. I'm not sick. I'm not dying. What are we going to the hospital for?" Inside, I was shaking like a small child who's been dropped off at preschool on the first day.

By now I was lucid. My parents had been instructed by a doctor to have me admitted to the UNM Mental Health Center based on my very obvious symptoms and severe psychotic state. I, without a doubt, had bipolar I disorder. That information was, of course, either kept from me, or I completely denied and ignored it.

My dad got lost, and we ended up at the main UNM hospital. With some help from a police officer in the parking lot, we "successfully" found our way and soon pulled into the Mental Health Center. Hmm, I thought. That's funny. Who knew God would end up at the local Mental Health Center? Well, whatever. I'll just go with it.

My parents checked me in at the front desk. There were no set appointment times. Nope. First come, first served. We waited in the lobby forever. And there were a lot of people to be served on that May 24 in 2001—it must have been a full moon.

I was paranoiac and really agitated while waiting my turn. I remember lying on Mom's lap trying to rest, but my damn brain would not stop thinking. I was really frustrated, spewing out every word that entered my mind. I didn't know how my physical body had been able to keep that speed up for a week. I felt like my brain was running a race. I had so much planning to do to save the world, which is why I was so agitated. I kept telling myself, I just can't lie here. There's so much to do.

Then there was the paranoia. People were staring at me, getting a really good look at God—me—to make sure they would remember my face because they knew I was here to save them. And for me to save them, I had to submerge myself in their world and blend in. Like an undercover cop.

Finally, my turn came to submit to the basics of temperature and blood pressure. "No blood," I said. "I'm God. I don't have any blood. And I don't have any veins, so you can't draw blood. I survive on air, like a fish. I have invisible gills that take in oxygen."

The nurse was calm and nodded in agreement to what I was saying. She seemed less than impressed (I guess she sees a lot of Gods). I didn't tell her I was here at the Mental Health Center to let the patients know that everything was going to be all right. They would be healed. I just had to lay low and follow protocol before I started applying my healing magic.

I was next sent across the hall to see another nurse, who asked me the same questions. I thought I was being interviewed so when the press showed up she'd have information to share with them. I was sure of it. I had much to share with her, so I talked as fast as I could. The more the press knew, the better my plan to spread the good news to the masses. It was coming together beautifully. Meanwhile, my parents waited in the main lobby—in hindsight, a huge mistake. The second nurse sent me on my way down the main hallway—alone.

I headed off to Financial Aid. The second nurse had told me where to find it (oh yeah, like I could understand directions, much less follow them). Halfway down the hall I took a right hand turn—and waited. Again. Well, at least I got there. When my turn came, I explained that I was God and that the paperwork really wasn't necessary. The sooner I could talk to the patients, the better, I said. Well, they weren't particularly moved by my speech, so paperwork it was—just like the common folk.

Okay. Bring it on, I thought. I signed documentation that said, yes, on this day of May 24, 2001, God arrived at the UNM MHC. Apparently, God took the form of a woman to make the arrival less obvious—and no, I wasn't dressed in a white robe, just shorts, a t-shirt and brown, flat, open-toed Jesus sandals. I had wild hair and no make-up, which probably explained the stares I got from people.

I'm right-handed, but with a pen in my left hand I scribbled "God" on each form, not caring to read any of them. "Let's just hurry this process along," I complained. "Oh, screw the paperwork. Honestly, is this really necessary?"

Not much was said from the other side of the glass counter, except I was asked to wait—again. Talk about trying my patience. Even being God made that challenging. My parents found me and we waited together. They became Jesus and Mary, and they were there to protect me. We were a team and with them by my side no harm could be done to me.

I went to the restroom around the corner. When I didn't come out after a while, Mary, my mom, came to check on me: "Michelle, are you okay in there?"

Sometime between leaving my seat in financial aid and entering the restroom, I decided that clothing was no longer necessary. We've gone back to Adam and Eve, I thought. And Eve didn't eat the apple, so it's okay. We don't need to be ashamed of our bodies.

DIAGNOSIS

My mom called for help from a nurse and between the two of them they tried to convince me that yes, I did need to keep my clothes on. But I wondered about how was I to set an example of being completely free if I wasn't showing it myself? They were both freaking out while I was laughing hysterically about the whole situation. I also decided women should be free and that bras weren't needed. I flushed mine down the toilet, but fortunately my mom reached in the toilet and snatched the bra just before it disappeared from sight.

Proclaiming my introduction into this "earth school" was not looking like it would be an easy task. And I thought Mary would be happy to hear about the no-clothing-needed-any-longer rule I proclaimed. No way. She didn't believe anything I was saying or doing. I was so high in my manic state I wasn't making any sense to anyone. But in my imaginary world, all was well. I was well and here on earth to share the good news with the world. People were slowing down—stalling. Not ready or prepared for my arrival, or so I thought.

Sometime after registering as God and proclaiming the end of the need for clothing, I managed to take a little journey down the main hallway of the hospital, clueless to where I was going. Another sign for me being at the hospital was the chaos that erupted when a loud siren went off. I thought it was the fire alarm. And I thought people were going to knock me down as they darted out of the building as fast as possible, but luckily they recognized my Godly appearance and ran around me.

You'd think the place was on fire with all the rushing, scared eyes, quick breathing and stomping feet. To me the scene was happening in slow motion. I continued my wandering and ended up in someone's office. The people inside asked me why I was there. I repeated my story, once again.

I really needed to get out a press release, I thought, so I wouldn't have to keep repeating my story about who I was and that everything was going to be okay. I thought with these inspiring words people would relax and want to talk and be around me. No way! They ran from the office like I had the plague. Oh, well, I thought. Each to his own. That's not going to keep me from moving forward with my mission. I rooted around in the office. I was curious. I found a box resembling a lock box and opened it. Inside was the most hideous looking thing—a toilet paper holder with colored ribbons hanging off both sides.

What in the world? I thought. "It's okay, people," I yelled. "I've found the pipe bomb. This is what set off the alarm. It's okay. It's not real." I examined the paper holder. "Who made this thing, anyway?"

A police officer grabbed the object from my hand and immediately started asking me questions. "What's your name, Miss?"

"God."

"Do you go by any other name?"

"Yes," I replied. "Michelle."

"Okay, Michelle," the officer asked with pen and paper in hand. "What are you doing in this office?"

"I don't know. I was just walking around. Everyone was running because of the siren, but I don't see what the big deal is. I found the pipe bomb, which was only staged.

"Yeah, let's frighten everyone with a make-believe drill so they'll be prepared for the real thing. Kinda sounds like the boy who cried wolf. Know what I mean?

"Anyway, if people were thinking it was real then they need to be informed that I've come to save everyone, and I've disengaged the bomb with a simple statement 'There are no bombs, there are no wars, there are no weapons, and there are no fires, floods or crime.' Therefore, everyone in these jobs are free to do work they enjoy that is in line with my plans to create peace on earth."

The police officer escorted me to the front door of the hospital, where my sobbing mom was waiting. Neither she nor my dad knew where I had been. Looking for me, my dad and a nurse had gone around the back side of the hospital. Losing me was not a good thing. I could see the newspaper headlines, "God gets Lost in Mental Hospital." Oh boy.

My dad finally met up with us and was just as grateful as my mom that I'd been found and wasn't harmed— except by the fact that no one was taking me seriously. Geez, it was a tough idea to convince people that God was disguised as a woman.

We stood in the parking lot outside the Mental Health Center and watched as fire trucks and police cars entered the building. A little melodramatic, I thought. Too many ER episodes for these people. Who knows how long we waited outside. But I began to check out people's shoes. I really liked some of the women's sandals and told my mom she was my personal shopper and I was going to need lots of really comfortable shoes. I trusted her to keep me properly dressed while I was on my mission.

At last, the sirens ended and I was escorted down a long hallway by two police officers and some techs. I didn't realize that my parents weren't with me until I turned around to look over my shoulder. To this day, I remember vividly my dad holding my mom in his arms while she sobbed uncontrollably. It absolutely broke my heart.

I didn't understand why they were crying, though. Maybe they thought they hadn't protected me enough and I was going to be locked up for my own safety. Maybe they thought they failed to protect my identity and that being held in a mental ward would keep the press and others at bay. Part of me felt very, very sad—uh, oh sad. I didn't know why.

Suddenly, being God hurt emotionally. I didn't know God actually experienced hurt like humans did. It's a snapshot moment that I'll always remember. Maybe this was the beginning of when I knew my life would definitely not be the same.

But it was. Upon entering the ward, my role of God resumed. I was asked to have my blood pressure checked. Of course, I had no blood, I thought. Therefore, what was the point in checking my blood pressure? My temperature was also checked. God doesn't have a temperature, I thought. God never sweats, never freezes and adjusts to the climate automatically. My outlandish ideas blurted out of my mouth as soon as they entered my brain, like shooting bullets from a gun. I was ready and armed for whatever came to me: Come on boys. Whatcha' got next? Just try and test God and see what happens.

They didn't give up easily. I vividly remember standing at the front counter talking with one of the techs. Before I knew it, he and another tech, whom I didn't see, grabbed me by the arms, turned me around and took me into a room with a mat resembling a wrestling mat on the floor. Boy, was I ever wrestling for my life. Somewhere, somehow, two other men grabbed my legs and all four of them gently pinned me stomach down. One held my head so I couldn't move. They were much heavier than I. My mere 127-pound self had no chance against the force of these men.

I had nothing on my side other than my large lungs that screamed so loud and for so long I could've shattered windows. Every muscle in my body stiffened. They're going to rape me, I thought, and there are people outside this room with the door open and they're ignoring me. They're going to gang-rape me, impregnate me and leave me with some venereal disease.

I didn't feel like God, but I didn't go down without a fight. I was scared. Shit scared. I had never watched Cops or other violent shows. I had never experienced anything like that in my semi-sheltered life. I didn't do drugs, smoke or drink. The screaming reverberated throughout my body. I tried to lash out. I tried to bite the hand of the tech who was holding my head. I was flopping around like a fish on land, trying desperately to wriggle myself free from that episode that has remained tattooed in my mind.

There had been no warning—no explanation. No being escorted gently using both legs. It was simply, bam, grab an arm, bam, grab the other, and turn around. Step, step, step, grab the legs and place on mat. I must have missed dance class the day when the mental health strut was taught. They were courteous enough to not slam me on the mat, though.

As if that weren't bad enough, I turned my head slightly over my right shoulder and saw a tech holding a syringe in the air. "No!" I screamed, squirming and sweating. "Don't drug me. No!"

They're going to knock me out, I thought, so I won't move while they gang rape me. I screamed so loud, I could feel veins popping out of my neck. My hair was wet with sweat flowing down my face.

"Relax, Michelle," the syringe-holding tech said. "Relax your muscles. Everything's going to be okay."

"Like hell it is!" I yelled. "Rest my muscles? Yeah. Why don't you see what this feels like and let me know if you'd be willing to rest your muscles?"

With my adrenaline rush, anger and being more scared than I ever had been in my life, I had no idea how long this went on. I thought the four men were going to kill me. They were going to drug me, rape me and leave me to die on the mat: "One, two, three, she's down."

I couldn't take it anymore. My body collapsed and I gave up. The physical exertion had left me completely depleted. "Do with me what you will," I said. "You may have my physical body, but you'll never have me." I lay on the mat, panting hard with a dry mouth and sweat all over my body.

"That's it Michelle, just relax." The tech lowered my shorts slightly on my right side and raised my shirt slightly to expose the flesh.

I was motionless. He stuck the needle in my lower back on the right side. Prick. I felt the needle go in. I cared. But I was too exhausted—mentally and physically to fight back. I felt like a dying fish on a stream bank struggling for my last breath.

I lay there for a few minutes completely still. Three of the men left. The one holding my head stayed. My breathing was the only sound in the room. The tech asked if I was okay.

"My neck's stiff."

He let go and I lay there. I didn't move. I didn't think. I was just still. Breathe in and out, I thought. My heartbeat echoed in my head. The tech closed the door and I asked him to leave it slightly open. I'm afraid of the dark.

The room spun. I looked around for something to focus on. Blue equals heaven, I thought. Keep blinking and looking for blue. It's all around me. The color of the walls—baby blue. As soon as the blue would come into focus it would turn to black—black which equaled the color of death.

I kept refocusing my eyes and looking around the room for blue, but it always would grow and change into black.

DIAGNOSIS

My heart was beating so loudly it engulfed my brain. I can't handle this God, I prayed. Please help me. I'm really, really scared. I don't want to make a sound for fear something horrific will happen.

I drew up my legs and rolled up in a fetal position like a ball. I covered my ears and closed my eyes. Whatever was going to happen I was too scared to hear or see it.

AT THE HOSPITAL

"Don't walk in front of me, I may not follow; don't walk behind me, I may not lead; walk beside me, and just be my friend."

—Albert Camus

The smells of dinner—bread and other aromas—awoke me. Silverware clattered. I was suddenly aware of how hungry I was. My stomach began to grumble. When was the last time I'd eaten? No recollection. But I was definitely up to eating a full, home-cooked meal (okay, not even close to home-cooked, but it was hot, smelled good and I wasn't about to turn it away). While I waited for my "specialty meal," I lay down on my mat, faced the ceiling and yelled to whoever could hear me what I wanted for dinner. This was a catered event, right? I made sure they knew I was a vegetarian.

To make sure they heard my request, I bellowed several times about the various kinds of fish I'd like to be served, along with vegetables, rice, a roll and soy milk (I'm lactose intolerant). I made all this very clear.

A man guarded my door. He was one of the techs who had pinned me down. I wailed my menu request to him, certain he was passing the information on to the chef in the kitchen. They have *such* good customer service here, I thought.

My meal was delivered by a kitchen staff man. He set down my tray in the dark room, and I noticed my vegetarian request had reached the staff. I asked him if he'd like to join me. He politely declined, leaving me to dine by candlelight—mental health hospital style, that is.

I was starving. I ate everything. Then the combination of a full stomach and the shots I'd received made me very groggy. I felt like I was drunk. A nurse came and guided me to my room, which had a simple wool blanket tucked into a single bed; a small, brown bedside cabinet; cold, gray linoleum tile; and one window with a view of the courtyard.

"I'm not staying in this hell hole," I told the nurse. "Who the hell decorated this place? Where is Martha Stewart when you need her? No, this is all wrong. We need a beautiful fluffy, floral comforter with a canopy overhead.

"And for heaven's sake, what is with the cinderblock walls? We need to brighten up the place with some nice pastel color, perhaps coral or lavender and hang some lovely pictures on the walls. Everything is just so wrong here. I can't sleep in this room. It's like prison." Upon poking my head in the bathroom, I thought it was equally unimpressive.

The nurse showed me option number two—the original room where I was sent when I arrived. She turned on the light. The room was even more depressing than option number one: a gray wrestling mat and various clothing items in the corner. Were they *my* clothes? I was very confused, but I knew the military room would be my primo choice where I would stay for five days.

The first night I had a roommate who snored. I was pissed. I couldn't sleep. I stared at her. I sent her telepathic messages for her to stop snoring. They did no good. Eventually I passed out from a full stomach and the drugs in my body.

•••

8:00 AM. Clattering dishes. Voices muttering. The wafting aroma of eggs and syrup woke me. I wandered out, half asleep, rubbing my eyes, trying to orient myself with my surroundings. A cart had been wheeled in to serve us breakfast. I stood in line, wearing my mom's long pink nightgown and matching robe. I figured if the rooms weren't going to be colorful, at least *I* could be.

The phone rang and some guy picked up the receiver. "Yes, may I please speak with Michelle Holtby" said the caller.

"Michelle, phone call for you," the guy said, handing me the receiver.

"Really? Wow, who would be calling me?"

"Good morning, Michelle," my mom said.

"Oh, hi. Good morning, Mom. I was wondering who would be calling me here."

"How are you feeling?"

"Much better today," I replied with a sigh of relief.

"You sound much better."

"Yeah, I had a really good night's sleep. They're serving us breakfast now. We're having scrambled eggs, toast, cereal, juice and milk."

"Sounds good."

"I need to go stand in line. They're almost done serving."

"Enjoy your breakfast. Dad and I will be there to see you at 5 o'clock for visiting hours. Okay. We love you, Michelle."

"I love you guys," I replied. "Bye."

Boy, I thought. That was really nice of my mom to call and check on me. I don't know how she got the phone number, but it was definitely nice to hear a familiar voice.

I sat down with a group of patients. We traded food items—cereal and eggs—just like in elementary school. And the trading happened at every meal. Everyone was there for a different reason. Yep, we were quite a group. Compassion played a role among us, and a quiet understanding glued us together.

"You don't know what you've got till it's gone," the old adage says. Losing my mind is what it took for me to appreciate the simplicities in my life. And that hospital stay was the first time I ever had that feeling.

I called my good friend, Robert, at work, filled him in on the details of my hospitalization and asked if he would come visit me. "Definitely," he replied. Unfortunately, I didn't realize there was a 10-minute phone limit. I was gabbing and laughing on the phone for a half hour. The staff said they'd unplug the phone if I didn't hang up—immediately!

Robert, who I hadn't seen in a couple of weeks, called my parents for directions and he showed up shortly before my parents arrived. I felt like he was visiting me in my new "home." I showed him around and offered him some milk from the patient refrigerator—but he politely declined.

I had stayed up late—11:00 PM—the first night in the hospital and had written Robert a 12-page letter explaining what had happened with Warren, how it led up to me being hospitalized, and about my marriage plans once I got discharged.

I don't remember how much of the letter made sense, but I was relying on Robert to pass the information to Warren so he'd be ready to continue with our wedding plans. I trusted Robert and knew that I could count on him to be my liaison.

5:00 PM came quickly. I waited by the entrance to the ward for my parents and waved when I saw them—I was never so happy to see them. The episode reminded me of when I was picked up at preschool at the end of each day.

When he was done reading the letter, Robert tucked it in his pocket, just as my parents rounded the corner. Timing. It's a beautiful thing. I didn't want them to see it. I thought they'd crash and burn my plans to a glorious, romantic marriage with the man I loved (obviously I wasn't in my right mind).

The four of us sat down around a table with chairs that weighed so much, no one could move them. I guess they wanted to decrease theft or late night chair-throwing matches. Perhaps they value their chairs a great deal. Who knows? Well, at least they were comfortable.

We all had a good visit and enjoyed a casual conversation. My mom brought me clean clothes for the next day. The two hours went by too quickly.

...

I was really looking forward to seeing Warren again, and every day I asked the same questions: "Where's Warren? When is he coming to see me? Does he know I'm here?"

My parents replied that it was best I not be in contact with him anymore, which confused and enraged me. I couldn't get out of my hospital prison cell to talk to Warren to explain our future plans and to tell him that I very much wanted to marry him. I was anxious the entire time I was hospitalized, hoping and praying that he hadn't given up on me and had found another true love. For the life of me, I couldn't remember his phone number. And my parents weren't about to give it to me. Time and space and healing were my priorities during my five-day "mental vacation."

I kept asking my parents "Where's Warren?" each day they visited.

Their answers told me something was up: "He's on vacation" or "He had a family emergency." They had an inkling about the whereabouts of Warren, but they didn't want to scare or confuse me.

Ouch. I've never been broken before, granted, heart broken, but not the kind of broken that leaves your mind spinning and your heart racing with anxiety. I have an overall numb feeling. This is the kind of broken I'm talking about. Broken down, like a car, without AAA or a mechanic in sight.

Death is the closest analogy I can use to illustrate my world after I was diagnosed. It was like being stranded in the middle of the desert without water, food or communication with the outside world. This was accompanied by the endless pounding heat on my head, and the burning into my skin the words "bipolar disorder." No, there was no way out of my "desert" for a long, long time. The first year was unbearable.

How cold and matter-of-fact can someone be when matters of the heart and mind are at their most extreme vulnerability? Perhaps a lawyer during trial, but a patient, me, just receiving the "death sentence" of being diagnosed with bipolar disorder?

My attending doctor, while I was hospitalized at the UNM Mental Health Center gave me the good news that after five days in the incubator (mental health ward), that I was being discharged.

"Oh hallelujah! Thank you, God."

For the first three days when my parents came to see

me during visiting hours I was positive that I was a permanent resident. How would I get my snail mail? My e-mail? I craved communication with the outside world. "Help! I'm suffocating."

Contrary to my hallucination/delusion of being a "permanent patient," my parents assured me numerous times that I'd be returning home soon.

"When? Tell me? I need proof!"

Approaching the front desk with wild eyes, and hair to match, I wanted answers.

"Why am I really here?" I had convinced myself that I'd merely had a nervous breakdown from excessive stress and being locked up here in this "mental hotel" was doing nothing to make matters better.

Everyday I approached the front desk wanting answers "When am I going home?"

I would check the clock every hour on the hour waiting for my parents to arrive for visiting time.

"Is today the day you bring me home? Please, oh please. The food here sucks, I miss my bed, my soft, fluffy comfortable bed, my room. How did I get here? This is just a great big misunderstanding with lawsuit written all over it. I want my life back. Besides, I have an interview with a radio station in two days as a sales rep., so work with me here people."

My parents, psychiatrist, medications and time were my core existence.

"If I don't make it out of here by May 27th I'm going to be homeless. No job, no money, no home." More Adavan, please. My anxiety level is rising faster than an elevator going to the top floor.

My parents daily visits were my one saving grace during my week as a lab rat, I mean patient (or consumer, as we're officially called because we consume mental health services—medications and psychiatrist appointments.)

We talked about daily, "outside-world" activities that kept my brain engaged. *Real* conversation. This is what I craved. It kept me going each day. I would reflect on our conversations, carry them with me, like a memory bag, and pull them out as needed.

They were my lifeline from day to day. They helped me cope with my negative mood swings when my self-esteem was gone and I didn't feel I had hope for *any* kind of future. These memories were my "pillow" of hope that comforted me. Through the anger, sadness and anxiety, the memories were right there, never fading away. Never letting me lose hope. This pillow, these good memories, were God taking extra special care of me. Protecting and comforting me.

· · ·

It wasn't too much of a battle giving up my title as God. I was actually quite thankful. The stress was unbearable. As I learned, *believing* in God is much more productive and easier than *being*, or in my case, proclaiming I was God.

For seven days and six nights, God was there with me. Through the tears, the pain, the frustration and the fear. He was there. Before my hospitalization I never really had a strong belief in God, but for me, it took this tragic event to relearn how to pray—a lot.

It shouldn't take a tragic event for me to revert to the ultimate "911 call," but it did. God hears prayers and it was a fast and clear reply. He was there for me and I had my parents. But all of my friends had vanished, except for Robert who hung around long enough to see me discharged and then exited from my life.

I can honestly say that being in the hospital ward was *more* terrifying to me that being able to pursue my manic freedom. The other patients, the environment, the daily blood draws and sleeping alone in the dark. It was hardly what I'd call a mental vacation. It was all new to me and it was really scary.

This wasn't my world, as I watched a young anorexic woman walk by me with a walking I.V. attached to her arm. I cringed. She was so rail thin all I saw were her bones. She was a walking skeleton, barely even existing. If I touched her I felt she'd crumble to pieces before my eyes.

Ironic, I felt like my life had crumbled, completely collapsed—overnight. The only difference was this was the vivid picture in my mind. On the outside, I was a healthy looking young woman who was in desperate need of a shower and a hair brush.

"I can't believe we need to get permission to check out razors and combs. Okay, give me the form so I can sign it. How ridiculous is this, I thought to myself. Never during my six day stay at the hospital did I think about physically harming myself. I had "scary hair" going on and wanted to look somewhat presentable. And not shaving for five days—I was just about able to French braid the hair on my legs.

I raised my leg up on the front counter to show the staff that I really did need to shave. I figure the more proof I could provide, the better. I felt like a kindergartener asking the teacher for scissors. I felt like saying "I promise to behave and use it the proper way and return it to you when I'm done. Scouts honor."

Oh, I got a razor, all right. A dulled one that I could've flossed my teeth with (but I didn't.) I guess they had multiple users of this razor that I received with utmost gratitude.

"Oh, you behind the desk most holy of hospital staff, thank you for granting me my wish to shave my legs. And how shall I repay you?"

Honestly, I looked worse physically when I was discharged. But at least I was rested and started on proper medication. My brain felt better and I was glad no one saw me for several days after I returned home.

The humiliation was too much for me to face. I needed a bag to put over my head. "Mental illness—oh geez. How am I going to explain this to people?" I thought over and over as we made our way to the car. My mind was caught in the spotlight and I was speechless. I wanted to hide— forever. I felt like an embarrassment and disappointment to my parents. I wanted to crawl into bed and not show my face again until I'd "gotten over" my mental illness, like an emotional flu.

LIFE WITH BIPOLAR DISORDER

"All you need to do to receive guidance is to ask for it and then listen."

—Sanaya Roman

After five days, I was discharged. I felt better and more myself. Fortunately, I had been given the right meds and correct doses from the beginning, and the meds kicked in quickly. I thanked the staff and my doctor, said goodbye to my inpatient friends and, with a lump in my throat and a small smile on my face, left the west wing of the Mental Health Ward and returned to the real world.

• • •

I had been protected living in my little cocoon world at the Mental Health Center. Quiet. Safe. Small number of patients. Every need was taken care of for me. Cooked meals were served three times a day at exactly the same time, there was plenty of time to talk with others, read, and watch TV. (I caught up on Oprah). And I had made my bed.

Yes, even though it had been a drab, plain environment, it was my mental "bed and breakfast" for five days.

Upon returning home, the first thing I did was call Warren. No answer. I drove by his house, but he wasn't home. I went to the park that evening, anxiously awaiting his arrival. He never showed up. I walked around and around the park with Tigger until it began to get dark and both of us were dizzy. With some confusion, I eventually gave up and slumped my way back to my car, seat-belted Tigger in and drove home with tears falling down my face like Niagara Falls.

Not hearing from someone, I realized, is much harder than hearing from them and having them explain why they don't want to be a part of your life anymore.

...

It was several months—six, to be exact—of black-hole loneliness. I returned to my home to be alone with my thoughts and Tigger. Numb. Not blinking. Not capable of thinking. Zombie-like existence. Wandering around my house, looking at laundry to be done, desperately needing to dust furniture, removing cobwebs and layers of dust and dirt from the weeks gone by.

I honestly think if someone had poked me with a pin I wouldn't have felt it. My life was constant sadness, crying for hours, and sitting for hours and doing nothing. No one to talk to. But, thank goodness, Tigger, the caretaker of my heart, was there to ease some of my sorrow. I began dialogues with myself. Being an only child, I was used to talking to myself, so it came quite naturally to me. Another way to escape, I thought. The conversations started out like echoes:

"Hello...hello...hello...how are you...are you...are you?

Where are you...are you...are you?" I started to think I was at the Grand Canyon. I stopped the "monkey mind" buzzing in my head, sat on the cold and hard wooden floor in the living room and began doing yoga breathing—my one saving grace from two years of experience. I calmed my body and mind together by focusing on my breathing.

"Tick, tock." I heard the clock on the wall but I wasn't bound by time. Time ceased to exist. The downward spiraling into a hole of pitch black darkness made me forget everything. Nothing I thought or did had any meaning whatsoever.

Damn, I thought. Is this what a nervous breakdown is all about? Shit! I'm only 27. I'm way too young to be experiencing this. The doctor claims I have bipolar disorder and all along they've misdiagnosed me. Lovely, just lovely. I'm taking meds for an illness I don't even have. I thought my psychiatrist would know the difference, but because I'm young they probably ruled out my having a nervous breakdown. But who says what age you can or can't have them?

Well, screw them. Screw all of them! I'm determined to bounce back from this setback and prove them all wrong. I'm going to be exactly who I was and do exactly what I did before this misdiagnosis.

With that, and a metaphorical sword of steel with a mind to match, I was on my way to conquering the world—to pick up where I left off prior to my diagnosis. I could feel it. I could picture myself being successful, getting along with co-workers, being involved in extracurricular activities after work. That's what I thought life was about—fitting in, conforming to the norm—a rat race world.

I couldn't *wait* to return. What I thought was productive, forward thinking mentality, however, was really me running tapes in my head over and over about the past. I even rewrote the bad parts to give them a shiny new coat, like applying wax to a car with dents.

I was determined that going back to work would be my second chance. It was my second chance all right, a second time to fall back into my black pit of doom when I started hearing voices—voices that were not exactly cheering me on to pursue the life I once had and would never have again.

The book is closed, the voice said. Locked and put away forever, Michelle. There is no looking back—especially now. Your pain is too fresh, your emotional wounds are pounding with their own heartbeats, crying out for answers.

After hearing the voice in my head, I replied, "So you're telling me that everything I did and said prior to this bogus bipolar diagnosis was for nothing? I busted my ass to make lots of money, to please people I didn't truly like, dated people to not be alone emotionally or physically and obsessed about the world I was creating for myself? All of it—for nothing?" Whoa. This is so not what I want to hear right now—and especially from a voice in my head.

I fought back. Okay, what else ya' got? Come on, sock it to me. I'm ready to fight. I've got my boxing gloves on. Come on. Show me your face. Or are you too chicken to reveal yourself to me?

Oh, Michelle, the voice said, it's not like that at all. I'm sorry I've upset you so much. In time, I hope you'll come to understand that everything in your life prior to your diagnosis did and still does have significant meaning. But to move forward with your life required a drastic change, like a train coming to a complete halt and throwing you off—something so shattering it would leave you empty—like being reborn. You're beginning to create book two of your life.

Book number two? I countered. Now you're sounding

like Bible talk: the word according to Michelle.

Well, something like that, the voice said. You're kind of on the right track. Over time you'll see how the puzzle pieces will come together to create a life that is God-centered—not ego-centered.

Whoa, what are you talking about, ego-centered? If I'm correct, I thought the whole purpose of anyone being placed on earth is to accomplish things.

Yes, that's true, the voice continued. But where this motivation comes from determines what kind and type of life you'll live. Believe me, you are not alone here. The only difference is that you were rescued from a life of eternal unhappiness, loneliness, frustration and confusion.

Wow, I replied. And to think I'm in a bad spot now.

Yes, Michelle, I see right through your sarcasm, and as I explain and reveal insights over time in your thoughts and dreams, I hope you'll learn to like and trust me. And yes, I realize that trusting—or even being willing to listen—to a voice in your head is the ultimate step in the right direction to begin your book number two. Consider it your New Testament according to Michelle or "In Michelle's Voice."

Okay, so now what? I asked.

No—not "now what." Just sit. Wait. The most important thing is to remain open. Trust your heart. Try not to think too much about what's happening. Analyzing things will only lead you to confusion.

MEMORIES

"The future just ain't what it used to be."

—Yogi Berra

Christmas 2001 was the bleakest, saddest holiday season I'd ever experienced. I was newly diagnosed with bipolar disorder the previous May and I was trying to grasp the sense of what living with a mental illness was supposed to be like.

The year was becoming bleaker as each December day inched by. Everything Christmas-related made me cry, such as carols played on the car radio, Christmas lights and yard ornaments decorated around the city, and even TV commercials for the latest "must have" gadgets. Storming out of the room in disbelief at the TV, I'd scream, "I refuse to watch this crap! Who honestly finds love and peace in giving these gifts?"

I felt as if I was losing my mind and I'd never see the world the same again. One message rang loud and true for me this year—Christmas was not meant to be celebrated by the mentally ill.

How could God give me this illness? Me. Successful, independent and confident Michelle. God, I thought, why did you strip away these positive qualities that took me so

89

long to build up? I was going somewhere with my life. This isn't fair. I didn't ask for this illness. Not now! Not ever! And so tell me, how exactly am I supposed to put the "merry" in this year's Christmas?

I was numb, hopeless and felt like a complete loser. What do I have to be thankful for this year? I have absolutely no idea. My health sure isn't at the top of the list, I said sarcastically to myself. And I'm only 28. How sad is this?

Why, God? I wondered. Why did you give me this illness that's destroying my life? The life I built for myself that took so long and, in an instant, you removed it all. It's not fair. I want a redo! What did I do so wrong to have to live the rest of my life with a mental illness? I'm sorry. Please. Let me try again. I beg you, I'll be better. I'll do better. There's got to be something I can do to make my life right again. How am I supposed to return to any kind of life I had prior to this God-awful news that is becoming more real and more nightmarish with each passing day?

My diagnosis turned me into a recluse or as I liked to call myself, a "bubble girl." My "cocoon" (home) was the only place where nothing or no one could harm me— mentally or emotionally. I was very fragile and the smallest thing either sent me lashing out in hostility or crying like a raging river. I decided it was best for everyone that I just stay in my cocoon. It was like being in a womb. I learned that I needed quiet, solitude and the warmth from the sun to keep my inner monster under control. My meds hadn't been regulated yet, which didn't help at all. I felt helpless. I felt like a science experiment.

Reasoning with myself, I tried to convince myself of God's goodness. I came to the conclusion that He wouldn't do this to me. It must be the devil at work. I'm so sorry God, I thought. What did I do? Reverse this and make it better. I promise I'll live my life according to your plans...not mine. I'll even go to church every week. I promise.

...

It was really weird how walking around with a mental illness felt like I was wearing it on the outside for everyone to see. My secret was being broadcast to all as my mom and I made our way through a shopping center during a busy December holiday afternoon. Christmas carols blared in the background as if the sound of familiar holiday jingles brings out the generous spirit in all to purchase, purchase, purchase!

I thought I was going to be nauseated. I had no money and definitely no Christmas spirit in my heart. Is this what a mental illness does to a person? I wondered. The lump in my throat returned with a burning rage. Let the tears proceed, I thought. No, wait! Not here. Not now. I've got to keep it together so I don't embarrass my mom. I may be a complete wreck, but I have to keep looking normal. The tears will just have to wait until I get home, or at least to the car.

I swallowed hard and forced myself to focus on my feet, a coping technique I learned from my therapist. As the music pulsed its way through my body, I kept tempo with each step I took, forcing myself to breathe normally.

I was getting anxious. The blaring music, people talking and babies crying was too much for my new, sensitive self to cope with. I used to be able to handle this just fine, I thought. What's wrong with me? Staring at the back of my mom's shoes, I followed her lead. She was on a mission. And I was along for the ride.

"It'll be good to get out of the house and get some fresh

air," she said.

I sure hope she's right, I hesitantly thought.

"Michelle, let's stop by the Christmas store." My mom looped her arm in mine, smiling at me. "I want to get some custom ornaments made for some friends. You know them. Remember, we went to visit them in '85? They now have three little ones and her sister has two little ones."

I wanted to scream at the top of my lungs, "Will someone just shoot me now?" I managed only a low-level "Okay."

"When did Christmas become all about kids?" I asked my mom. "What about dogs? We should get a special ornament for Tigger. He *is* your grand-puppy." And the best thing I can give you that's closest to a grandchild, I sadly thought.

I gulped hard. Ouch! I hate that burning raw feeling in my throat, I thought. It's like a bomb that's been lit and is sizzling inside my throat. I feel nauseated.

So many words wanted to flail out, like projectile vomiting. And I knew they would—in their own time.

"What do you think of these ornaments, Michelle?" my mom asked, holding two matching snowmen side-by-side.

"They're fine," I said nonchalantly. As I looked at the snowmen, I wondered, is this Christmas? These ornaments handmade in China with names carefully printed on their bellies?

I felt empty and sad as I watched the associate carefully print each letter with such care. I wished someone would print my name on a happy holiday ornament. Perhaps it could have improved my mood. I wanted to feel important, too—not that it would have changed anything. I would have probably thrown it out of the store or smashed it, but it would have been a nice gesture.

"I'll wait for you outside, Mom" I managed to say,

quickly darting out of the store.

As I leaned over the handrail, I gripped on for fear of another round of tears breaking through my emotional dam at any moment. I was like a time bomb, experiencing emotions I never knew I had and with such intense levels. Anger, resentment and confusion were the top three *that* day.

While my mom paid for her purchases, I noticed she also bought the ornament I had selected for Tigger. I tried to collect myself and appear as a normal shopper. I looked around at all the people. I wondered, are they really happy? How much stuff do people honestly need? Our society is taught that stuff equals happiness. No wonder there's so much debt! I thought this realization would make me feel better, but it just left me empty.

Speaking of which, I thought, how in the world am I going to pull off Christmas this year? Buying nice gifts for my family and friends had never been an issue before. I prided myself on being able to pick out just the right gifts for my loved ones. They were always chosen with care, wrapped and received well and with love. And of course, working in advertising and earning a lot of money meant even nicer gifts. Expected and selected. It was automatic.

Of course, in college, I was forgiven for not having money to spend on lots of gifts. My grades were gift enough. But once I hit "Corporate America" things changed—and I was expected to change right along with them. Success equaled money, and money equaled gifts, and gifts represented love. Yes, I fully believed this and lived it for five years.

From the burning sensation coming from the balls of my feet, I guessed my mom and I had been at the shopping center for a couple of hours. What was I thinking, wearing boots to go shopping? Oh, well. At least I could focus on a physical pain to keep my mind off my mental anguish.

Our last stop was a high-end gadget store that sold everything to make life easier. Walking inside, I did not get this feeling. What I got was sticker shock that left me with an overwhelming sadness. I just stood and stared at various items that people I knew would love as gifts, and in return, they would love me. One of the "affordable" items was $49.99. Yeah, right, I thought. Where am I going to get the money? Donate plasma? Pray for a money tree to grow in our backyard? Who am I kidding?

No one even approached me to see if I needed help. I must look sick. And poor, I thought. I sensed the workers seeing my bipolar germs dripping off me onto the floor. I took a shower. My clothes are clean. Oh, I get it. I don't have that "glazed-doughnut, gotta have it" look in my eyes.

I couldn't see my reflection, but my whole being felt sad and lethargic. I felt old and tired. I was fighting an unfair, unwanted battle with no weapons or energy to help me. You know what would be great? I thought. A bipolar disorder survival manual. Wonder if high-tech land sells them? Maybe they'd have different levels:

1. Welcome to the Newly Diagnosed (a.k.a. the end of your life you once knew)
2. Keep on Trucking
3. Living Well, Staying Well

The manual would totally make my Christmas, I surmised, as something helping me and not band-aiding with temporary things to mask my pain. No such luck. I don't see a single book in the store.

Perusing the store, some golf items caught my attention. My dad loved to play golf and he had a business trip coming in January. I spotted a great, travel-sized golf game that was perfect for him. I got so engrossed in the product and testing it that when I saw the price of $49.99, my eyes immediately began to water.

Then my dam broke. "I can't afford this. I can't afford crap!" I cried to my mom. "I'm used to giving you and dad nice thoughtful gifts and now I have this stupid illness and I can't buy, do or say anything right anymore. When are things going to be right for me again?"

"Shhh, Michelle. It's okay." She handed me a tissue. "Here. Blow your nose."

I sobbed into the tissue with my back to the door. "I don't care who's watching us. I can't take this pretending everything's okay when it's the farthest thing from the truth.

"I want to get dad this travel golf set, but I can't afford it. No one even offered to assist me, to see if I had any questions. Yeah, here's a question. Why is your merchandise so damn expensive? Is it made of gold? It's probably good they didn't approach me. I was feeling hostile and the last thing I needed was to be escorted out by security."

"If that's what you'd like to get him," Mom said, "that's fine, Michelle. You can pay me back later."

"Okay." I blew my nose and went to the cashier.

"Would you like this gift wrapped, ma'am?" asked the employee with an overly cheerful smile.

You damn bet I do, I thought, and there better be gold flecks in that wrapping paper. "Yes, please, that would be nice."

Mentally counting my steps to the car, I could feel the burning, lit bomb in my throat begin to rise again. It was on fire. The tear faucet turned on and, without shame or guilt, I let the tears fall and run down my jacket. My mom and I didn't speak. I thought getting my dad his golf gift would help elevate my Christmas spirit, so *why* did I still feel a raw, empty feeling inside?

I was certain that all my parents wanted for this Christmas was for me to get well. Me, too. But, unfortunately it wasn't like having a cold. You don't take medicine for five to seven days, then return to feeling better.

Bipolar disorder goes on and on, month after month of taking medication, year after year, with the sufferer praying for no repeat hospitalizations. It's a debilitating lifetime illness and I didn't have the first clue how I was supposed to live with it. It was my nightmare that I carried around with me—always a reminder I was "broken" and there was no turning back to the life I once knew and loved and worked so hard to create.

That life was gone—overnight.

ACUPUNCTURE

"Genuine beginnings begin within us, even when they are
brought to our attention by external opportunities."
                                        —William Bridges

It had been just over a year since my diagnosis. I felt
great in part because I had the privilege of receiving
massages once a month. During one of my sessions, I
told my massage therapist about my menstrual cramps and
how they'd been getting increasingly worse as I got older.
She had seen a Chinese acupuncturist for a similar condition, and she recommended him because her symptoms
disappeared after several treatments.

Acupuncture sounded like an answer to my prayers.
My cramps got so bad I'd vomit from the physical pain. I
suffered from constipation, my lower back was so tense I
could barely stand to touch it, and I got bloated, which
usually lasted for three days. I got anxious each month as
time grew closer for my period to start. My periods were
absolutely horrible and after trying a number of things, including teas, homeopathic remedies and prescriptions from
my doctor, I was more than glad to try something new.
Something had to work.

I visited the acupuncturist shortly after receiving the

referral. I was glad he could see me the same day I called. We talked for a while and after I described my symptoms, he told me to change into a robe and he'd be back in the room in a few minutes.

I had no idea what to expect. My palms were sweaty and I wiped them on my robe. It was two weeks before my next period would start. I figured there was plenty of time to see how well my body would respond to acupuncture. I looked around the room. There was a poster of the male body with chakras and meridian points on it. I remember learning about them in yoga. Man, there's a lot of meridian points, and I forgot what they did.

The diminutive acupuncturist came back. He motioned for me to get up on the examining table. While clutching my robe, I saw he was holding a small tray with at least 100 little needles standing upright.

I gasped. Okay, calm yourself Michelle, I told myself. They're only needles. I could feel sweat beading on my forehead.

He set the tray down by my feet where I couldn't see it. I think it was better that way. He started talking to me—just a general conversation—and then the needling began. Having never experienced poking by a needle other than shots in my arms and my ears when I got them pierced, I was not prepared for the jolting pain when he jabbed one in the inside of my right ankle bone, then in the top of my foot.

"Crap! That hurts," I said. "I have *no* fat on my feet. Why are you putting needles in my feet? I have menstrual cramps—there are no feet involved." I sat up on my elbows to examine what he'd done to me. I was beginning to feel like a voodoo doll.

Somewhat panicked, I asked, "How many more of these needles do you need to insert?" If all of them were going to hurt like that I was seriously considering exiting stage left.

ACUPUNCTURE

My poor ankle. It reminded me of when I was 5 years old and got my finger treated for an infection. The doctor who treated me didn't prepare me at all. He just grabbed my chubby little hand, held onto my index finger and dug out the gunk that had formed a "home" next to my fingernail.

I'll never forget how long and how loud I wailed in his office. And when the receptionist asked if I'd like a lollipop on the way out, I stated "NO!" in the most pissed-off 5-year-old voice I had. How amazing it is that childhood memories can arise from our current situation.

After five days of visiting the acupuncturist I was feeling great. Thankfully, my body had adjusted to the needles rather quickly. He didn't stop at my feet. He inserted them all over my body (in the meridian points, I believe). Fortunately, most of the needles had soft landings into tissue on my body, so I didn't feel a thing.

But *no way* did I let him go above my neck. I don't know what it was, but something just totally freaked me out about having needles placed in my neck, face and top of my head—sorta' like a porcupine. Just the thought of them made me cringe.

Every day I went for treatment it was the same routine. My mind soon got over the fact I was turning into a human pin cushion. I think the fact that the acupuncturist talked to me during the entire procedure greatly diminished my anxiety of the needles. I don't know exactly all of the benefits the needles had, but each day I felt better—much better. I was more relaxed and laughed more easily. I wasn't experiencing "monkey mind" for the first time in a very long time. It felt like my body was being recharged from the inside out.

I was feeling so great that, on my own, I decided to stop taking my psychiatric meds. I went cold turkey. I had been taking four prescribed medications for the past year and they were working well, but I didn't think they were nearly as effective as one acupuncture treatment. On day two of my treatments, I announced that I decided to stop taking one of my medications. The acupuncturist looked concerned and asked me why I would do that.

"I feel great!" I said. "I feel more alive and energized. I didn't even need a nap yesterday. This acupuncture stuff works fast—and it's all natural. I'm tired of dumping more chemicals into my body. Who knows what they're doing to my brain."

"Hmm, I don't know about that," he said. "Did you check with your doctor before you started doing this?"

"Are you kidding? No, I'm perfectly capable of taking care of myself and as long as I feel good then everything's okay." But it seemed that nothing I said would console him. "I saw the sheet in the lobby that lists all of the ailments that you treat. Depression, anxiety, PTSD and paranoia were on the list. I don't know why bipolar disorder wasn't." I just thought he forgot to include the disorder, so I let him go at that.

Each day I was more "high" than the previous day. I was like a balloon rising in the sky—floating higher, getting more manic and not caring where I ended up. I felt free and light and with no responsibilities. I'd felt this way before and I loved it. Why couldn't I hold on to this feeling? I was like a child with endless energy. I was so happy I never wanted it to end.

•••

I told my parents at dinner on the third day that I'd been seeing an acupuncturist for my menstrual cramps—even though I wouldn't know if or how well his treatment

ACUPUNCTURE

worked for another week. I said I discovered that he also treated bipolar disorder. My parents looked at each other with raised eyebrows and panic in their eyes.

"Relax, guys. I know what I'm doing," I said.

"Are you taking your meds, Michelle?" my dad asked in a concerned voice.

"A couple of them. I've been reducing my meds each day I go in for a treatment."

"Did he tell you to do that?" my mom asked anxiously.

"No, I'm a big girl. I made the decision all on my own. Why keep dumping more and more chemicals into my body when I'm being cured through acupuncture?"

"Michelle," my dad said, "acupuncture is not a cure for bipolar disorder. It's very dangerous for you to stop taking your meds. If you keep this up you'll end up back in the hospital."

"Yeah, whatever," I said. "I feel great. So, why do I need pills? I might as well be taking placebos. It's been over a year now, I should be cured of this bipolar thing by now, and if I don't want to take my pills there's nothing you can do about it. I would think you'd be proud that I'm trying to find a solution to this illness so I can get on with my life."

My dad didn't know what to say. My mom started crying.

"I don't know why whenever I talk about my illness everyone gets so bent out of shape. I'm doing what's best for me. Can't you see that?"

"Michelle," my dad admonished, "you're going to end up back at the Mental Health Center if you keep going down this road of not taking your meds. This is very frightening and sad for Mom and me to see you go through this again. Surely you remember what it was like when you were taken in a year ago and got diagnosed and hospitalized."

"Yes, I remember," I said. "It was a misdiagnosis of a nervous breakdown and this will prove it to everyone that I am fine and do not have a mental illness! Why doesn't anyone believe me? This is like a really bad made-for-TV movie.

...

As my parents predicted, after five days of acupuncture treatment and my reducing my psychiatric meds daily, they readmitted me to the Mental Health Center with another acute phase of mania. I was God again and I felt great.

I had a rapidly increasing mania that included thinking I was being followed by snipers who could see through our home. Armed with rifles they were out to capture God (me). Tigger was safely put in the sunroom. My choice.

The hospitalization in mid-August lasted only three days. I was not cooperative about taking the meds the nurse dispensed. I resented the fact that no one believed that I'd had a nervous breakdown. Pills were *not* the solution to this problem, I thought.

I was summoned to court to determine if I could be released to go home even though I refused to take my meds. I thought I was hallucinating. There's a courtroom at the Mental Health Center? I wondered. Okay, whatever.

I thought my imagination was continuing to be overactive, so I just went along with it. But no, it was for real.

The courtroom is actually inside the hospital. I was on trial, after being there for only three days, to determine if I should be released to my parents care. I wasn't compliant on any kind of medication. I refused to take what I had initially been prescribed—but I don't remember why. I think it had to do with denial of having bipolar disorder. I was so determined to go home, I hardly said anything. I felt like a mannequin on display, breathing ever so slightly so as not to move a hair on my head.

My heart pounded out, "Oh, please let me go home today. Please let me be released." Surely, I thought, the courtroom could hear them.

It felt like a movie. I was given an attorney to represent me. My parents, the doctor, the judge and I were present in a very small courtroom. I felt like I was on trial. Every single breath and movement I made was recorded. I felt if I blinked wrong that I'd be back in the ward, so I remained as still as possible. I wanted out of the hospital and this was my one chance to achieve my goal.

I could play the angel they needed to see—anything to get out of this place. I don't remember saying anything in the courtroom. My court-appointed attorney escorted me into the hallway near the end of the trial and asked me some questions to see if I knew what was being discussed and if I felt well enough to go home.

I nodded. Yes, I'm going home today, I thought. Oh, thank you, God.

With a big smile on my face and a bounce in my step I reentered the courtroom. The judge said I had a right to refuse medication and there was no evidence I posed an immediate threat to myself or others. I was granted permission to go home that day. It didn't take me long to pack. I'd traveled light on that journey. I said good-bye to the friends I'd made and gave hugs and encouraging words.

My parents talked to my attending doctor and waited for me in the courtyard. I looked through the glass in the door and saw their angst. They did not look happy. I didn't understand. I thought they'd want to have me back at home. Oh, well, I figured they'd get over it and things would soon get back to normal.

EXPLOSION OF ANGER

"Be careful what you ask for, you just might get it."

—Anonymous

I t was a pleasant evening at the dinner table—until World War III broke out.

"Of all the people in my life, I would think that you both would understand," I screamed at my parents. "You honestly think this is some sort of vacation I'm on? A Carnival Cruise, perhaps? Believe me, I'd much rather contend with motion sickness than this eternal illness. Yeah, I just woke up one day and asked God to spice up my boring life.

"Okay, Michelle, here you go," God said. "Not only will I spice up your life, I'll completely spin it around so fast you'll wonder if you're dead or alive." My mind flashed on "ask and you shall receive."

"You couldn't be farther from the truth," I continued. "This vacation you seem to think I'm on—well, I want to tell you IT'S NOT A FUCKIN' VACATION! It's a life sentence I was born with and which came alive at my young age of 27. You think this is fun? I beg to differ.

"By all means, feel free to whip out the party favors and the band. And don't forget to invite your friends and family. Yes, let's celebrate the fact that Michelle is no longer a successful career woman with a good job and a home owner with a steady boyfriend. What a great joy! My ass, a great joy.

"You just don't get it. I look well on the outside, appear to act normal, and you forget that I'm sick at all. Surprise! I'm NOT WELL! I'm in remission, but my symptoms can flare up at any time, like a dragon getting ready to breathe fire on its enemies. Do *not* mess with me, especially about the few weeks that led up to my diagnosis."

The memories of my past were still raw, like a bandage being ripped off and exposing a bloody, oozing gash for everyone to see. It's painful and ugly and makes me nauseated. I can't stand to look at it, yet I must. It's part of me and will be, forever.

"I'm fully aware that I'm hypersensitive. Every little thing sets me off. I read more into things people say, mainly from both of you. Your words reveal hidden messages, a secret code that is spoken to me by God whenever you talk to me."

My parents had idea what was going on. I was having flashbacks and hallucinating. The messages from God were very helpful and assured me that I was on the right path, following His directions until He returned to earth. I was His secret agent again. I didn't know if there were others like me who were chosen to be God's secret agents, but I wasn't going to share that with anyone. It was huge news and I feared ending up in jail.

I now know I experienced post-traumatic stress disorder (PTSD)—not reserved just for those returning from war. I vividly recall the time I spent with Warren. I mentally relive it, just like watching a sad, old horror movie— only there's no popcorn or candy. (Tears and tissues, please.) The movie's in color and stereo surround sound.

EXPLOSION OF ANGER

The color blue equals "good" or "God" and black equals "evil" or "the devil."

I also experience transference where some memory from my past leaks its way into my present life. And, sometimes, the bad memory gets cancelled out, like my caring, kind and trustworthy friend, Pete, who replaced the manipulative and mentally-ill Warren. And some memories, like my former boss, have been replaced by my current boss.

But honestly, why me? Analyzing things doesn't help. I'm uneasy and I can't breathe. My anxiety medication does little to calm my nerves. I can't focus on anything for longer than half an hour. Anxiety becomes my world and until my angst is resolved, I am not me. I hate the month of May.

The anxiety in my body makes me sore when I wake up each morning. My jaw is tight from clenching it all night. My muscles are stiff. My left hip joint hurts. I feel like I'm 100. It hurts to walk. My feet are tight. I wiggle my toes and circle my ankles listening to the "snap, crackle, pop" as they go around and around. Why can't I just relax?

I feel "on" all the time. My mind doesn't rest. I'm always thinking about something, mainly reliving a prior negative experience, over and over, letting it resort to its comfortable downward spiral, like a spaghetti noodle going round and round a fork on a plate. Sometimes I catch myself and sometimes I don't. It's the *don't* part that scares my parents. I don't give a rat's ass. I want revenge.

"Do NOT tell me I'm depressed because I lash out in anger at you for all the crap that's occurred this month," I said. "I'm stressed out to a 10-plus and you want to what? Call my psychiatrist? Like hell you will."

"When do you see your doctor next, Michelle?" my dad said. "Michelle, when do you see your doctor next?"

I turn my back to him, mumbling, "I don't know. Next month."

"I need to speak with her."

"Like hell you will!" I yelled. "I'm 30 years old. I can take care of myself. Depressed you say? You have no idea what's been going on these past few weeks. You never seem to want to be around to talk to me about things.

"Oh, let me take that back. When I'm doing well, all is well with the world, but the minute I become upset, you bail. You leave the room or tune me out. Who are you? You didn't act this way when I was growing up. You always listened and were there for me. What's changed?"

The recurrent burning sensation in my throat gave way to a nonstop stream of tears. "My problems are very real and important to me and having you block me out kills me. You don't care anymore. Where's my dad who was always there for every stage of my life when I was growing up?

"I may not know how to be deal 'effectively or appropriately' with anger, but here it is. Deal with it. Suppress it? I think not."

All this only makes me angrier. I feel like pulling off my head and shaking it like a coconut to let whatever wants to come out to do so. Just pull the cord at the base of my skull and let the screaming festival begin. Ooh, look at the steam rising around me, my red, flaming hair dripping wet. My red eyes probably appear as if I'm possessed by an evil force. I am Michelle! Hear me roar.

Such a sweet, young lady people say. This can't be her. Hah! Meet Dr. Jeckel and Ms. Hyde, otherwise known as Michelle's bipolar disorder at its worst.

I continue ranting. "And why is it that I'm fine when I'm out in the world, but feel stressed out and anxious when I'm at home? Gee, maybe because you're both the source of my anger and are here to receive the bullshit I've had to deal with these past few weeks. You don't want to hear it? That's just too damn bad. I don't want to live with this bipolar disorder thing anymore. Care to change places? You'll get to experience just how 'fun' this vacation is you seem to think I'm on.

"Everyone expects things from me. Why can't I just be? I'm losing control. Everyone's pushing me into situations, into fulfilling their needs. My happiness is being compromised. It's feeling like my advertising jobs all over again. What didn't I learn then that has to be repeated? It's killing me inside—mentally and physically."

I was losing my happiness, I thought. I felt like everyone was taking it away from me. Sucking the life out of me. My joy. My very essence.

How and when did I let this start happening? I wondered. I can't breathe. Not even my chill pills ease the tightness in my chest and my throat. I'm shaky—inside and out—as if someone has put me on vibrate mode. I can't sit still. My mind has not rested for three days.

This is *not* good.

•••

The Mental Health Court judge appointed my dad as my medical legal guardian for six months following my release in August 2002. Every few weeks he accompanied me when I met with my psychiatrist. Gradually I returned to taking my medications because I realized the fact that I did have bipolar disorder and there was no way out of it. For the majority of an entire year, anger and rage tormented me.

This was *not* a good time for me, or my parents.

DBSA-TELEPHONE
OUTREACH
COORDINATOR

"Make your own recovery the first priority in your life."
                                        —Robin Norwood

I remember when I was first diagnosed thinking this was the absolute *worst* thing that's *ever* happened to me. "This isn't right. It's not fair. I'm too young to have my life ripped out from under me."

I tried to recall all of the horrible sins I'd committed to lead God to this decision. I came up with a few, but they were from my high school days and I figured I'd long been forgiven for them. Elementary school didn't count, we were too young to know right from wrong.

"The end of my life has arrived. I will never do or be who I once was. I'm broken—forever."

I remember sitting in a chair at my parent's house and just crying, for hours. About what? I do not know. I was numb. It was too much to process. The tears flowed freely down my cheeks. I felt a sadness I'd never felt. Alone. No one to share my emotional pain with. My parents didn't understand what I was trying to explain, my psychiatrist, who I saw once a week listened to the story of my moods and made medication changes accordingly. This did little to console me. I felt like a science experiment.

"Am I getting better yet?" I thought to myself. It felt like the same ol' turnstile every six months with a new doctor. Fortunately, I'm blessed with the ability to be very articulate and although I couldn't concentrate long enough to read or write even a paragraph, I knew what I needed and I knew how to convey it to my psychiatrist.

Two words "chill pill." My saving grace. My daily escalating anxiety episodes leave me paranoid, fidgety, feeling "on" constantly and unable to control my negative downward spiraling thoughts. This anti-anxiety medication smoothes over the anxiety bringing me back to the present moment, where I want to live. It helps me relax, like having a cocktail or a beer—only there's a lot less calories and no hangover—and you don't have to be 21 to take it. Daily afternoon naps and my "chill pill" are the two constants in my life now.

...

Back to sitting in the chair in the sunroom. Eight hours have passed by. I hear my parents car turn into the driveway. I don't budge. Kleenex and several days worth of mail surround my feet, proof that I actually did breathe and am still alive.

"I don't care about anything or anyone. I want and need comfort and it's unfortunate that the one person I can turn to–God, I don't.

"I've lost everything with this damn diagnosis. Gee, let's count the ways: I was fired from my job, I had to sell my home because I didn't have any money (and didn't win the lottery in time), the few friends I had have vanished. And let's not forget the additional losses of my sanity, self-esteem and dignity. How in the world can anyone prepare for something like this?

"Yep. Without any notice at all, I gradually crept up to the hypo-manic phase in about two months and then BAM!! I was blown through the roof with an acute manic phase of bipolar disorder."

Warnings are good. But what's a warning when you have more energy, need less sleep are creating more ideas and are overtly social? Sounds like an extrovert to me.

I love analyzing things. How and why did I get this horrible illness? I'm determined to figure out how I got it and then work my way back to get out of it. To move on with my life and never look back. This isn't like a bad case of the flu. This is like being diagnosed with cancer, only instead of chemotherapy and the high probability of being cured, the best we bipolar people can pray for is to reach "remission" with medications, psychiatrist visits and managing our stress level.

"I'm so ashamed of myself. This isn't me. I want answers."

After about six months of daily crying spells lasting for hours I begin to emerge from my protective "shell." I tell my psychiatrist I need some answers. I'm craving knowledge, like putting puzzle pieces together.

"Books. People. Please. Whatever it takes, I'm willing to learn. No, I need to learn everything possible about this illness to survive."

"Please help me understand it," I ask my psychiatrist with pleading eyes during one of my weekly visits.

"It's killing me inside. I hate not knowing what's going on with my brain and I resent the fact that these little pills you prescribe me aren't doing squat. When are they going

113

to start working?" They may as well have been placebos for all I knew.

•••

"Well, Michelle. There is something you may be interested in. It's a support group that meets here at the hospital once a month. It's called The Depression and Bipolar Support Alliance (DBSA.)

"Yes, keep talking." My ears soak up the information my psychiatrist shares with me. This is good.

A tiny start to crawling out of my aloneness cocoon. I've never been in a support group, but I didn't hesitate to go at all. My mom was great. She offered to go with me. I felt intimidated in this foreign support group land.

"Do I really belong here? Do I have to qualify to be "sick enough" to participate in the meetings?"

I remember the first meeting I went to. It was at the hospital. The president went over some announcements, we wore name badges, went around the room introducing ourselves and personal information, had a snack break and broke into two groups—one for depression and one for bipolar disorder.

Looking around the room I felt incredibly out of place. "I'm the youngest one here. I'm not going to have anything in common with these people. It feels weird being here. I don't know how I'm supposed to open up to these strangers and share my private thoughts. That's what my psychiatrist's for."

I remember everyone was in their 40's and 50's and I felt like a misfit. But, I kept going to the meetings, along with my mom. I mainly listened, but just being there among a group of my peers was somewhat comforting.

Several months later, the meeting place got moved to a

nearby church. DBSA is non-religious based, but moved because there were several larger rooms to accommodate the support group's growth. And the rent was affordable.

I'd attended meetings for about a year and finally began to relax and talk to some of the members. I was still one of the younger ones in the group, but as time went by, age didn't matter to me. I realized we were all in this bipolar thing together and sharing our experiences were what bonded us together, ultimately helping us to heal.

There were usually 10-15 people who attended each week and it became a comfort for me seeing these same people. I eventually got brave enough to share some of my personal life with a few people. I won't lie. It wasn't easy for me at *all* to open up to a group of complete strangers, but once I did, it was a great relief and release of resentment, tension and fear. It's not a twelve step group. Although there is a trained facilitator and each person has an opportunity to share with the group whatever's on their mind.

Camaraderie comes easily for me. Bipolar disorder affects every age, race, sex, educational and social-economic level. No holds bar. *"So, why me?"* I would continue to ask myself this question for *many* years to come.

After being a "regular" at these meetings for a couple of years, I was approached by the DBSA president after one of our meetings. She asked if I'd be interested in doing telephone outreach. "Sounds interesting. So, what would I do exactly?" I asked. I didn't know what I'd be getting into. "Can I handle this?" as hesitation resonated throughout my body. I hadn't "worked" since my diagnosis. "What if I fail or give the wrong advice or get completely overwhelmed?

"We get a lot of phone calls each week from consumers as well as from parents. They want to know where they can get help. They want someone to listen to their personal stories. You'd mentioned that you'd worked as a telemarketer and I think this would be a good match for your skills and DBSA's needs. I haven't asked anyone else yet, but I hope you'll consider helping us out.

"I'll pray about it and let you know my answer at next week's meeting. Wow! Who would have guessed? My first volunteer job. Well, it seems like it would be a good fit." Driving home from the night's meeting with a grin on my face, I knew what my answer would be. I looked forward to being able to give back to DBSA for all it had given me. The next week I accepted and I was off and running, to where, how and who, I did not know. But, it felt right, so I just went with it.

Like at my MCI telemarketing job ten years earlier, I was uneasy at first. I didn't know *what* to say, but hoped I helped the caller in some way. I had a script and over time it got modified and answered all the general questions newly diagnosed people have about DBSA and how to cope with their loved one and outreach that's available for them.

I can honestly say, it was the most rewarding thing I've done with my life so far. To be able to give back to others what wasn't there for me. I couldn't have been at a better place or time. I provided comfort, DBSA meeting information, and I believe a sense of hope with each caller. By sharing my personal story with these callers, who were complete strangers, there was a connection through the phone lines. It was like a comforting word blanket to calm their nerves to help them accept and embrace their worries, fears, frustration and unanswered questions.

For those family members who were seeking solace, I referred them to the National Alliance on Mental Illness (NAMI) for their Family to Family class. This is a free 12 week course addressing family issues with their recently diagnosed loved one, be it depression, bipolar disorder, schizophrenia, schizoaffective disorder, generalized anxiety disorder (GAD), obsessive-compulsive disorder and other phobias. Passing along this information to these family members made it seem like I'd given them gold. Only, this "gold" was answers to their prayers—absolutely priceless.

Nothing prepared me for what I agreed to take on. This was a brand new position and an opportunity for me that left me with unexpected gifts of empathy and reaching out to help others. I can't recall how many people I helped during the two years I was the telephone outreach coordinator, but my ability to listen, empathize and find good "matches" for solutions to each caller's challenges was the most rewarding thing I'd done with my life so far. I had purpose. I felt God driven. Who knew that a part-time college job could turn out to be such a good fit in this new world of mine?

...

So, what *does* happen behind closed doors at a DBSA support group meeting? Well, everything talked about *is* confidential; however, I'm willing to share what I talked about during my 2 ½ years with DBSA.

As I mentioned before, the first six months I was pretty quiet. Not quite knowing what to say, if it would be "accepted" and "relevant" for the group to hear. As I got to know some of the people, I became more comfortable, let down my guard and let my worries, anxieties and frustrations slowly come out of the dark and into the light where I felt freer at each meeting to share my thoughts and feelings. It was definitely a huge part of my healing process.

What my psychiatrist didn't have time to explain and what my parents didn't know the answers to, DBSA filled in the gaps. "Yes! This is where I belong. This is what I've been searching and waiting for, yet not knowing what I was searching and waiting for. Thank you God, once again, for answering my prayer."

I talked about my fear of weight gain, the effects of my medications on my brain and in my body. Feelings of personal loss, disappointment to others (mainly my parents). I received nods from others in the group. Being just a "new be" to the group, pretty much everything I shared was greeted with a "been there, done that" response. What a huge relief. Knowing that we were all in this together and I had an entire room full of people who were ahead of me in their recovery process. My mentors. My friends.

I felt like I was "home." Friends and family who didn't know *what* I was experiencing didn't bother me so much because I knew there would be relief at the next meeting, which was just one week away. Like a drug addict in recovery, I kept returning. These people were my lifeline to keep me afloat during these beginning stages of bipolar disorder—level one.

•••

During my four years as a DBSA member, my healing process gradually increased. I began to feel stronger— emotionally and mentally and therefore better able to address and handle my problems. It was one of the most crucial steps to my recovery process.

Now

BY YOUR SIDE

Five years, could it be?
Something wonderful is happening to me
You've got a hold of my heart
And given me a brand new place to start

I seek You in the morning when I pray
And I ask that you be by my side all through my day
You help keep me focused, and my heart open and free
And allow me to see it's with You, I should be

I've reached a point
Where I've discovered
The whys and ways
Of how to recover

What does healing look like?
How will I know when I've "arrived?"
The answer, so clear, so simple
When I feel most alive

When I'm able to give back
In various ways
I will know what I'm doing

Because it will sing God's praise

To sacrifice and share with others
Is what it means to recover
You've led me where I need to be
You've taught me how to be free

It was not easy
It took turning off my brain
And turning on my heart
To listen to You, God, from the start

I've shed my old life
There's no turning back
God, with you
Is where I'm at

I seek Your guidance
And comfort to heal
Please show me ways
That are true and real

May these words reach others
And be shared for miles around
For with You, God
Love, comfort and truth can be found

By Michelle Holtby©2008

PETE

"The words that enlighten the soul are more precious than jewels."

—Hazrat Inayat Khan

Santa Claus is coming to town. Believe me, I thought, this is one thing I sure as hell didn't wish for. It amazes me to this day how many Santa Claus clones exist in Albuquerque, and it bothered me immensely after I was discharged.

Santa's twin, he sure was. Every time a Santa clone approached me out of the blue, I felt as if I were jumping out of my skin. I imagined them saying, "Boo! Caught ya, Michelle."

Yes, I still get physical reminders of Warren, but I just breathe and remember what happened. I realize the clones are *not* Warren and I release any pent-up anger and resentment inside me. I chose to forgive him, but it took me four years. I came to a point of acceptance and forgiveness—with myself and Warren—at a spiritual retreat a couple of years ago.

It was the most healing, revealing experience I've had thus far in my life. I realized three very important things:

123

1. Warren was only human.
2. He wasn't mentally well.
3. He was trying his best to protect me from harming myself, but he ultimately drove me to a full-blown manic episode.

Ironically, he was the worst thing and the best thing in my life that month of May 2001.

...

Wow! 2001. Only four years ago. It seems like a decade ago. And have I grown. I drive by Warren's house occasionally, and whenever I pass by I remember to breathe in and out deeply. It's like holding my breath under water until I can safely resurface at the other side. Fortunately, I've found an alternate, somewhat out-of-the-way route to avoid his house and still get to places I want to go. I incorporated the route in my maintenance plan to keep me balanced.

Note: Each year, in the month of May, I refuse to drive past Warren's house when the memories rush in, and the anger, hurt and disgust about how I was used surface like uncontrollable waves in the ocean.

Honestly, out of all the men that God could've sent my way, why did it have to be Santa Claus' twin? If I had had my choice it would have been Richard Gere. He would have done quite well, thank you. The whole weeklong move-in thing probably would've been more enjoyable, too. But I suppose God thought about that also. So, Santa Claus it was—beard and stomach and all. Gross. Please don't try to get too vivid a picture of this in your mind. Vagueness will do just fine.

Fortunately, God helped me to see that not all men are like Warren. It wasn't until two years later that I met a man

PETE

quite the opposite of Warren. It's so true. And I'm so thankful he's in my life. I definitely know we're in each other's lives for a reason(s). Having him in my life is making my life's journey less painful and more enlightening and peaceful.

I wish everyone could have such a good friend.

And here he is. Come on out, Pete. Don't be shy.

...

Pete. My dear friend, Pete. I've never met anyone like him. He's amazing. He's kind, generous, open, honest and caring. Sounds like, well—me! We tried to make a go of it when we re-met during golf lessons two years after my diagnosis. During the beginning golf class lesson I saw him walk over to the putting area, and I did a double take.

No way, I thought. Oh, my gosh! I was so happy to see him again. We'd known each other a few years earlier through dance lessons, but it wasn't more than casual conversation. This re-meeting was like a "take two."

We both took the class for fun and we had a few more lessons together before the class ended. I pretty much stunk at golf. Let's just say the LPGA Tour was nowhere near seeking me as a new recruit. So we laughed and talked and hit golf balls all over the place while chucking up a fair amount of grass. I loved every minute of it.

We showed up Saturday afternoons from 1-3 PM, and I really looked forward to it. It was like an unofficial date. It wasn't a crush. It wasn't love. I finally figured it out about a year later. He was my *friend*. My very first true guy friend. Okay, okay, truth be told, we did date for a few months after golf lessons ended. It felt like we'd picked up where we left off from our first time dancing.

Pete's about a decade older, but when we spent time

125

together it didn't matter. We shared a lot in common and it was nice just being in his company. I felt safe. It was the first time I'd experienced that with a man I dated.

He was gentle and kind. What could I do? I shared things with him, bit by bit as time went by. I was drawn to him, gradually, like a magnet increasing in strength. Our phone conversations were great. He was a good friend and a good listener and supporter. Now, he's one of my main Wellness Recovery Action Plan (WRAP) support team members whom I completely trust with my life. (Note: I discuss my WRAP plan in the next section.)

It's amazing that he knows absolutely everything about me and still wants to be in my life. He is a true friend. Thank you, Pete, I often think, I never knew what a true friend was until I met you.

Pete helps give me peace of mind. He understands me and he has an amazing ability to empathize with me. He's my "go to" friend whenever I'm in crisis mode (any situation that greatly upsets me, such as arguing with my parents). The pattern for the past three years when I get really upset about something is to have a good long cry in my room. Then I call Pete and tell him what's going on. Somehow he's able to decipher through my crying what I'm saying. He never judges me or tells me what to do. He just listens objectively and gives me great advice and support. He always knows what to say. I am truly blessed to have him as a friend.

Several months ago he told me that my rebuilding of my life one day at a time was like making a movie. I never thought of it that way. Some people let life just happen to them. I'm more of an Amelia Earhart flying a plane over the Pacific Ocean with a map I can't read. And I'm afraid of heights, but I'm ready for any adventure with my co-pilot Tigger in the passenger seat.

PETE

I'm usually up for change, but not very spontaneously. I enjoy living and being free, with nothing or no one holding me back—such as my mind chiming in with "No, you can't, Michelle. You have no money and you have no one to go with." Those thoughts still live in full color in my mind. Sometimes they win and sometimes they really win.

But when they don't, *that's* when I'm living. That's when I'm "me" and when I want to socialize and try new things—even alone. That's when I feel confident and happy. Some may call that a hypo-manic stage. Perhaps. But it's controlled by my meds. And having good friends like Pete helps keep me in balance.

HUD HOUSING

"Often people attempt to live their lives backwards: they try to have more things, or more money, in order to do more of what they want so that they will be happier. The way it actually works is the reverse. You must first be who you really are, then, do what you need to do, in order to have what you want."

—Margaret Young

"Oh, my gosh," I said. "If I don't get out of here I'm going to go crazy!"

I'd been living at home with my parents for four years. It was time for me to have my own space. Looking back, I guess it was a sign that I was getting well. My psychiatrist sparked the idea during one of my sessions to encourage me to take the steps of moving forward with my life.

I was fortunate to be an SSI recipient after applying for it during my second year of disability. It was the only way I was able to afford low-income housing. I never thought I'd be disabled and I thought I would, like most people, reach the age of 65 before receiving Social Security. It was a matter of good timing, prayer and getting my paperwork turned in to the right people that expedited my applications, both

129

at the Social Security office and the HUD office.

I felt great after being given a voucher at HUD that told me how much I could afford as rent on an apartment. It was my ticket to freedom and moving forward with my life. I felt physically and mentally prepared to take a huge step and get my own apartment. The budget number looked so big on paper, and images of a beautiful environment entered my mind, which made me smile. By the end of day three, after searching several sites within my budget, my smile was gone. I was stressed, drained and anxious. I thought it was supposed to be fun. The places I was shown were so unimpressive. I guess my middle-class lifestyle left me with higher expectations. The biggest lesson I learned: it's expensive to live. And I was supporting only Tigger and me.

The apartment complexes I had visited were as expensive as a home mortgage payment. I wondered, how in the world do people make ends meet and survive in this city? I couldn't believe the low quality of the complexes I was seeing. Martha Stewart, where are you?

The available units reminded me of my hospital environment, with one exception: I would be given a key to come and go as I pleased. The amount of time, paint, furniture and money it was going to take me to bring my potential apartment up to my expectation made my mind spin and tied my stomach in knots. I kept asking myself, is this really worth it?

After picking up a local apartment guide at the grocery store, I made a list of things I was looking for in my ideal rental: pet friendly, a security gate, two bedrooms/one bath, washer/dryer, centrally located, a small yard, quiet neighborhood, a garage, good daytime lighting for writing, and preferably a newer development furnished or unfurnished. It didn't seem like it would be rocket science for me to find these things and it shouldn't have been—it's called being a homeowner. My voucher was specifically for an apartment rental. Hmm, I thought, slight problem here.

After a week of dedicating myself to finding the perfect place, I crawled back home with my head tucked down, like I'd been beaten by society. Ha, ha, Michelle, my mind said. You can't survive out there in the real world. You're disabled and you're broke.

I've always been really good beating up on myself—one of my traits I'm not proud of. I never told my parents what I'd done. I wanted to look for my own place to live on my own. But more importantly, I wanted to show my parents that I could survive on my own with a mental illness, and sign a rental agreement, buy some furniture and move forward with my life. I also wanted my own place so I could have a place to invite friends and potential boyfriends over. Being 31 years old and having a guy pick me up for a date at my parents' home seemed so high-schoolish.

After moping around the house for a week, I made a decision. The voucher had an expiration date. I decided to turn my voucher back in so that someone else could use it. I knew there was probably someone out there whose living situation was worse than mine. It felt like the right thing to do. I never looked back. Never had any regrets. I knew when the time was right, I would move. Until then, having my laundry done, having food in the fridge and having the comforts of my parent's house would suffice just fine.

In addition to my apartment wish list, Tigger got to live dog-rent free and enjoyed a huge backyard, I got to take regular neighborhood walks with Tigger and my good friend, Gabby. I had everything I needed, and there was minimal noise.

I had to swallow my pride and realize that living at home again with my parents was only a part of my life, not the rest of it. I was looking at moving as a way to escape my problems at home. Moving never works, though. Problems follow us wherever we go. I have no doubt that another moving opportunity will come around. But for now, staying put is what feels right. And Tigger agrees.

OBSESSIVE-COMPULSIVE
DISORDER

"The worst thing that happens to you can be the best thing for you, if you don't let it get the best of you."

–Anonymous

When did the ritual thing start? I honestly don't know. I do know that it's grown to be quite an annoyance. Fortunately, no one else sees the unusual ritual things I do that keep me safe, like touching my bamboo plant in my room, bathroom, office and in the sunroom to give me good luck. I touch my St. Christopher medallion on my car's dashboard to keep me from harm's way when I drive.

I check or touch things multiple times. The backdoor locks at night are the worst. My anxiety flares up and I check them five to ten times on average before I fall asleep. Even with a house alarm, I'm still paranoiac the doors may not be locked. This has been going on for several years. I like to analyze things, and I believe this is a sign that I'm afraid to move forward, to trust, or to keep things out and away from my life. Whatever it is, it's an unwelcome part of my illness.

I consider Obsessive-Compulsive Disorder (OCD) to be a side order to go along with my bipolar disorder entrée. It's quite common and, unfortunately, my OCD symptoms have escalated over the years. And, like the seasons, they rise and fall from being acute to hardly there at all. They're really severe when my parents are out of town. I recently counted checking the door locks 12 times.

This is absolutely nuts, I tell myself. The doors are locked. The alarm is set. I can go to sleep now. It's like I'm giving my mind permission to rest. At times like these, I feel very much "on" and I can't rest until my nighttime medications kick in. Also, sleeping away from home I keep my eyes wide open and glued to the front door until my medications kick in. Whether I remain in the city or I'm away at a conference, the effect is the same. I don't do well sleeping in a different place. But that doesn't stop me from traveling. I anticipate the shift in my sleeping pattern, and I try to take a nap during the day to compensate. I also have my "chill pills" I can fall back on if I feel myself growing more anxious.

Like lulling a colicky baby to sleep, it can take up to an hour for my mind to be put to rest. I take a psychiatric medication at bedtime that slowly makes me sleepy, with the effect of descending in an elevator until I'm so groggy I can't keep my eyes open. I go to sleep and don't wake until the next morning. I've been taking the med for years and it works great, but I sometimes wonder if I'll ever be able to get to sleep on my own.

I've tested this question by staying up as late as possible a couple of times over the years to see if I could drift off to sleep without the aid of the nighttime medication. But the results were not good. The later it got, the more anxious I became. My mind started to rev up with negative thoughts, and it became hard to breathe.

OCD

What in the world? I never had problems falling asleep before my diagnosis, I would think. Why do I now? I have a concern that my brain has become dependent on a drug to help me fall asleep, but I suppose if it is what I need to get a good nine hours sleep, then so be it. Lots of Americans who don't have a mental illness toss and turn each night. I bet some of them wish for a magic pill to help them fall asleep—my wish has been granted.

I automatically attach special meanings to most of my lucky things. Just because I have a lucky bamboo plant doesn't mean I need to touch it to receive good luck. It sounds crazy and it is crazy. I can justify the rituals in my mind, but I just can't break myself of the pattern. Fortunately, the condition doesn't paralyze me or keep me from living my life.

I was reading a book recently that described the reasons people perform rituals. It said that rituals are performed "in order to create a safe resting place for our most complicated feelings of joy or trauma, so that we don't have to haul those feelings around with us forever, weighing us down. We all need such places of ritual safekeeping." The author goes on to say "that you are absolutely permitted to make up a ceremony of your own devising, fixing your own broken-down emotional systems with all the do-it-yourself re-sourcefulness of a generous plumber/poet."

While my OCD tendencies aren't full-blown rituals, they are, in my mind, an important part of creating balance and safety in my world.

In my office I have an "I let go, I let God" affirmation card on my computer monitor. I run my fingers over it while waiting for the computer to boot up. I have a lot of spiritual/healing/God-related objects to which I've attached meanings to keep me safe and have God continuously watch over me. I feel I have an extra dose of safety and protection from harm's way if I surround myself with spiritual affirmations.

In my bedroom I have a nightlight statue of Mary. Each night, after I turn it on, I rub her head before going to sleep. On my pillow, I also have a little cross-shaped pin, blessed by a priest, which I rub before I go to sleep.

And on my dresser, I have an altar that I created several months ago after I received a beautiful, inspirational card from a woman who knew me when I was in grade school with her daughter. It began with that card, which stays on my dresser to remind me to keep moving forward. It gives me hope and encouragement that I'm doing the right thing by stepping out and speaking up about my illness.

Then a second card arrived after Christmas last year from one of my dad's high school classmates. She had read my Christmas letter and was so touched she mailed me an inspirational card to keep me writing my book. It's also on my dresser. Eventually I plan to make a scrapbook out of all the articles, e-mails and cards that people send me. Either that or I should buy a bigger dresser to display everything on.

I believe that God is using me as a vessel to write this book. It's an amazing feeling to put pen to paper and let the words flow, bringing them to life and gracefully filling each page with color. This feeling isn't an OCD or a bipolar disorder thing. It's a very strong feeling I've had since I began journaling in my notebooks, where I let out my raw emotions on paper when no one else could hear me cry out in pain. It was such a lonely, dark time I'm thankful I had pen and paper to neutralize my endlessly streaming negative thoughts accompanied by mounds of tissues.

I don't know if I've always had OCD tendencies, and they were just brought out with my illness. Looking back to high school and college times, I don't recall me checking

OCD

locks and touching things for good luck. I remember I had a lucky pen in college that I used for blue book exams, but that's not so out of the ordinary. I also remember placing things in specific places in my apartment, but that was so I could easily find them. Perhaps these are borderline OCD traits, but I don't do either of those things anymore.

And finally, the newest edition—the eagle. My fixation with the eagle began when I read a book a friend gave me—before I was diagnosed—called *The Artist's Way*. In it, the author discusses different symbols and how everyone has a "land" animal and an "air" animal. My land animal is a green dragon and my air animal is the bald eagle.

The bald eagle is a good thing for me to see. It's God guiding me on my journey and it's a positive sign that I'm moving forward in the right direction. It goes beyond the physical animal, and it includes seeing it on bumper stickers, jackets, license plates, tee-shirts, titles or song lyrics, golf courses and even statues in people's front yards.

It's like a game to me. Several years ago, it used to surprise me when I'd spot an eagle symbol out of the blue. Now it happens regularly, and I may see the symbol once or twice a day. It's a reassurance that God is watching over me. I smile to myself and know that I'm being watched over closely.

And when it comes to making decisions, seeing the bald eagle will generally give me my answer, whether it's talking with someone or reading something. I'm not hallucinating. I can't because I'm on medication. It's more subtle. And safer.

But I feel a presence of God whenever I see an eagle. I'm not God. I'm not manic. I'm just Michelle having a connection with God. I believe that when I see an eagle symbol, or hear a song by the Eagle's, or hear the word eagle in lyrics, it is a symbol encouraging me to continue on

137

my path with God. The path that He has planned specifically for me: "Follow the eagle." While driving I may see
the eagle symbol on the back of someone's license plate, a
sign that I'm heading in the right direction. I don't stalk the
person driving in front of me, and I don't follow them to
their destination. The symbol's there to let me know that
I'm heading in the right direction. A smile always comes to
my face. I feel as if I'm being watched over by God—the
highest symbol of being connected with God.

EATING DISORDER

"Every problem has a gift for you in its hand."
—Richard Bach

"I'll be right back. I need to use the restroom," I say. I almost salivate as I eye the scale in the guest bathroom. My heart races. My palms are sweaty. I've got to know the number. What's the "magic" number that's going to make me happy or anxious? 135 Wow! Two pounds less from a couple of weeks ago. No, that can't be right.

Quietly I pull the scale back out towards me again, hoping the scraping on the tile won't catch Keith's ear in the kitchen.

135. Phew! This is great! This is going to be a great night. I feel light and happy—and sexy.

Keith *must* notice that I look *really good* tonight. It's a "high" for me when he says that I look nice or pretty, which in my mind means "I approve of you" and "I'm glad to be seen with you." When he doesn't say those things I feel insecure. I crave attention, perhaps it's the only child in me, and I'll do just about anything to get it. It's a "high" of a lifetime. Something that I'd developed a craving for since my eating disorder days began when I was 11.

"Wanna' see Michelle get attention? Watch her disappear, slowly vanish away? Yeah, there's nothing like dying to get people's attention." It's my control mechanism that I use when I feel I'm losing control of my life. Stay skinny. Be in control. It's as simple as that—for me, anyway. My fool proof plan.

I want to be the popular one chosen by a man. The center of attention. I want to feel *important.* I did my part, what's yours? It's always been that way with guys I've dated. Commenting on my physical appearance makes my heart skip a beat. He thinks I look great means we're going to have a good time tonight. He wants to look at something appealing and it damn better be *me!*

Keith's preparing a nice, quiet dinner for the two of us at his parent's house. Very sweet of him. He knows about my eating disorder, my anorexia, but not how well I hide it.

I quietly close the door to the guest bathroom. My heartbeat is pounding so loud. I recognize the "rush" of earlier times when the urge to know how much I weighed ruled my world. It was like winning at gambling.

"Oh please, don't walk in on me, Keith. I don't know how I'd explain this." I look fine. This is crazy! I'm over being tied to a number on the damn scale that rocks my world like a gambler or an alcoholic who takes to their vice.

I push the scale back out of view and take a good, long look in the mirror and say out loud "if I look good then he'll want to be with me. Be affectionate. Never leave." My inner cheerleader takes over center stage "He's not like the guys in your past. He likes you for you. Your intelligence, creativity, kindness, inner and outer beauty."

I want to believe myself, but somehow I can't. Not completely, anyway. Geez, I wish a new dress would remedy this situation, but unfortunately it's way deeper than that. I need someone to talk to, and I don't think Keith would understand. He's sweet and I'm sure he would try to be understanding, but these are some mixed up thoughts I'm having. And honestly, if he knew what I thought about myself and my weight I'm afraid he'd leave me. It's better and easier to pretend nothing's wrong. I say out loud to the mirror "Just go have a nice, quiet dinner with him, Michelle."

I feel like a shredded wheat commercial. Part of me can rationalize my way of crazy thinking and knows I don't need to "do" or "say" things to keep a man in my life. However, the other side relies on this sick, controlling eating disorder to get attention. Ah yes, attention equals love and this is what I'm truly lacking in my life. Not just any love—unconditional love. "When was the last time I felt this?" I think it was when I was a baby when nothing was expected, just eat, poop and sleep. When did life have to get so complicated?

But why can't a man just love me for me? Probably because I don't "walk the walk" and I have expectations from them. Is every relationship like this? Am I losing my mind? Will my anorexia ever be just a memory? 23 years have passed by and I still carry it around like a mental crutch.

•••

Then what's the *real* reason I feel this lack of control in my life?

•••

It's one week before my period starts. *That's* the connection to weighing myself. I don't want to grow up to be a woman. I want to remain a child. I'm pulling back. Retreating inward. I can't handle the "adult" world. I'm only

11. A child. I should be having fun, but instead I feel my life being taken away from me—my childhood, being ripped, pulled away from me.

"It's time to grow up, Michelle" I feel my parents pressure. But I don't start menstruating until I'm 13—7th grade. I have a best friend, but we never talk about it. It's too serious and mysterious. Too much "adult talk." It's too stressful. We just want to chase boys around the playground and talk about them constantly. I feel relaxed around them now. My body doesn't feel like it's the focus of my being—I can just be and they accept me for who I am. This was true until the boys begin to take notice of me later in the year. This was both a blessing and a curse. And 7th grade was only a beginning of my relationships with boys. To wait or to weight, that's the question.

"Dear God. I know one thing for sure; if I get pregnant my parents are going to kill me."

I know exactly what makes my eating disorder "tick." It's the same thing that sets my bipolar symptoms into full alert—stress. The more of it I'm under, or in, or experiencing, the bigger and faster the wake-up call to my one of three dysfunctional aids—bipolar symptoms, strictly regulating my eating or cranking up my obsessive-compulsive tendencies. The combination is enough to make me scream. And nobody knows. "She looks too normal. How in the world could anything be wrong with her? She's got so much going for her?" Well, let me let you in on a little secret, which I guess from this point forward won't be a secret any longer.

I'm scared to death of becoming pregnant. Yes, and I'm sure there are many women out there who share this same concern. But my being scared is rather sick and twisted. The *real* reason I'm scared to death of becoming pregnant is because I can't stand the thought of being fat for nine months and then having to turn around and work off the weight gain from the pregnancy. I'm afraid Keith's not going to be attracted to me any longer if my body shape changes and doesn't meet his expectations. I like the way I look now and having him repel against me would kill me inside.

My anorexia would veer its ugly head and come to the forefront to "rescue" me. Oh, I have no doubt I could lose the pregnancy weight, but it wouldn't be healthy and I'm afraid I would go overboard and lose more than needed, like an anchor being thrown overboard on a ship, only, I don't have an anchor and I don't know *when* to stop. I know me, and any kind of weight loss program would be an invitation for disaster. I wouldn't lose the "recommended" amount of weight; I'd push myself and see how low I could get the number on the scale to go. It's a game for me. A high. I salivate each time I step on the scale. My heart races. "Come on. Come on. Please let it be a lower number today. Yes!" Success. Only, my "success" would slowly kill me. I'm able to hide my eating disorder. It's sick and twisted and unfortunately, it's been with me since I was just a little girl. And it's not something that has a cure—only remission. Just like my bipolar disorder.

SAD

"The best-educated human being is the one who understands most about the life in which he is placed."

–Helen Keller

"Why me?" Just when I thought I had this bipolar thing under control this happily forgotten Seasonal Affective Disorder (SAD)
diagnosis, which I gave myself my freshman year during
the fall semester at NMSU, comes blaring back into my life.
Daylight savings time is not my friend this year—2007.

Five days. I'm going out of my mind. I'm so anxious
and moody and lethargic—and it's only November. I feel
like someone's taken over my brain. This is not me. I was
doing fine just 2 weeks ago. How could all of this come to
the surface so quickly?

I try grabbing on to anything to stop me from falling
farther and farther into a spinning cycle of flashbacks. I
can't turn them off. I've lost that capacity. I'm not that
strong. The memories surface like monumental waves with
never ending tears. I'm too weak. I don't fight off the
memories. My "chill pill" is back as a regular part of my
routine medicine plan. Something that's to be used "as
needed" feels like my life preserver. I've just *got* to hang

145

on until my SAD light arrives. I trust my psychiatrist and am thankful that she recommends the HappyLite™ by Verilux. She said I *should* see an improvement in about 2 weeks. Relief can't come soon enough.

Thank goodness. It'll be one week before Thanksgiving. Crying over a big, dead bird on the table with the family gathered around is *not* my idea of a good time. Especially since I can count how many times I've cried in front of people. Not something I'm proud of, especially since I consider myself to be so strong and independent. I'm good at fixing things and that's how I view my SAD situation. A task for me to "fix."

I ordered my Verilux HappyLite™ mini light system, I'm taking vitamin supplements, attend yoga once a week, a Reiki session once a month, a monthly massage and dancing (clogging and country) weekly. I *do* have a healthy balance of things in my life. But *knowing* the solution and *not* being able to implement it —waiting I do *not* like. It's frustrating to the point where I'm ready to put on my make believe boxing gloves and punch away the pain from my past—sometimes it's people I want to knock out and sometimes it's thoughts.

It's been 12 years since I graduated from NMSU and now my SAD symptoms are alive and kicking again. They're just as ugly and strong as when I first experienced them my freshman year. "Where in the world do they come from?" One day I'm fine, then overnight I feel like a completely different person. I can't even stand to be around myself. How in the world is anyone else going to stand to be around me?

...

Seasonal Affective Disorder (SAD). Crap! Just when

SAD

I've gotten a grip on bipolar disorder this thing resurfaces again. It's no surprise, really. The symptoms started during the fall term of my freshman year at college.

I felt depressed, but I didn't know why. I became weepy, withdrawn, and craved sweets and carbohydrates. I was lethargic and couldn't concentrate—a classic SAD scenario. When I diagnosed my condition after reading an article about SAD, I was relieved.

I didn't tell anyone because only six months of feeling "off" didn't seem so bad. I was sleeping through the night and taking a daily two-hour nap to make it through the day. I went to all my classes, completed my assignments and got straight A's. Living with SAD was going to be doable, I thought.

In the back of my mind, I knew that come spring I'd be back to my regular self. So, I just forgot about SAD and coped the best way I could with excessive sleep, isolation and plenty of chocolate—like a bear in hibernation with a sweet tooth.

Going home once a month to visit my parents didn't raise any warning flags that something might be wrong with me. My difficulties all took place at school, because that's where my stress resided—with classes, my room-mate and my environment. My home in Albuquerque was like a weekend retreat where I could escape—a place to catch my breath, sleep in my own bed in my own room, eat my mom's home-cooked food, have my laundry done and forget about classes.

It was a very lonely time for me. I missed out on so many social activities—football and basketball games, so-rority parties and hanging out with friends. I had no one.

As the days grew shorter, my mood grew darker. Al-most overnight I began to feel different. I didn't know who or how to talk to anyone about it, so I just kept my secret to myself.

I know I looked fine on the outside. I showered daily, even though I felt like a dead weight when I forced myself to the shower each morning. My clothes were clean and matched, even though it took me forever to make a decision about what to wear each day. There were too many choices and I felt overwhelmed. I was anxious from the time my alarm clock went off and my anxiety lasted every evening through dinner. My brain gave me a break in the evening, though, allowing me just enough energy to watch TV.

I was a walking zombie. I felt dead on the inside and it grew worse as the fall semester progressed.

I lasted only two months in the sorority. I couldn't handle all the "required parties" I had to attend. The last thing I wanted was to be around people. I just wanted to hide. And think of what to say? It was too tiring and I was overwhelmed. So I moved– the third time in four months.

Back to the dorm where I had my own room for the spring semester was a good fit for my symptoms. No required parties. Limited contact with my soon-to-be-ex-best friend, who was quickly drifting away despite being a neighbor. And, as an only child, having my own space was important.

I remember those nights when I'd see the stadium lights and hear the marching band play outside my bedroom window. But I had no desire to go out. I was content researching and writing term papers for classes. In my own way, I guess I did participate in those events from my "cocoon" by knowing the fun existed only a few hundred yards away from me.

...

The weather has been surprisingly warm through Sep-

SAD

tember and into October. It wasn't until daylight savings time hit in October 2007 that my mood changed—overnight with no warning. I had been doing really well. I know it's more than the temperature change. It takes everything I have to make it through each day. I refuse to let the depression win. Call it being stubborn.

I check in with myself. Is this the downside of my birthday celebrations? I haven't felt hypo-manic. I've felt balanced, doing a variety of activities each day, making sure I have plenty of down time. I'm taking my meds, eating well, exercising, going to yoga, and basically keeping my regular daily routine. Where did this drastic shift in my mood come from?

I'm very much "on" and aware of everything that comes out of my mouth. I don't want to say anything I'll regret and have to apologize for later. That takes too much time and energy, and I'm trying to avoid that at all costs.

How can I express how angry I am about something in my past without blowing up at a person? I don't know what to do. I want to see Keith, but every time we're together I'm afraid I'm going to say something to drive him away. But, he's there. He's my punching bag. It's not fair and I better figure out something to do before my anger ends our relationship.

Please, God, I'm lost. As I crawl into bed, I plead, "Please guide me." I don't know how or to whom to redirect my anger.

That's just it, I have no one to vent to. I don't feel God's presence. I don't feel like I'm getting help from anyone I talk to, even to Pete and Lori or my parents. They don't want to get in the middle of it, yet they see how miserable I am.

Why aren't you rescuing me? I wonder. How long can you tolerate me being this unhappy? I wish you'd tell me what to do. I'm failing at my relationship with Keith and I'm not a failure—not at *anything,* I say to myself. I'm a perfectionist.

"Yes, Keith is a good guy," I tell my parents, " but your first priority should be your daughter."

Why don't they just tell me what to do? I'm lost and broken and have nowhere to turn. I'm falling apart on the inside. And I thought the most important thing to both of you is that I'm happy and healthy. Well, hello, take a good look because this is so far from that!

Life seemed so much easier when I was a kid and my parents just told me what to do. No consequences, I suppose.

I'm really confused. Other couples must go through stuff like this. In the past, I'd resort to reading some kind of self-help book. I think I'm beyond that. I don't want to read. I want to talk. I want answers. Proven answers from people who will point me in the right direction.

Lori had it right when I spoke with her the other night. I asked her, "How do you know when enough is enough?"

"Michelle," she replied, "I think the question to ask is, "Do the happy moments outweigh the unhappy moments?"

I like this much better. I don't have an answer, but it's *something*, at least. Perhaps it's part of the answer to the equation.

I don't know how to effectively copy with my anger— anger like I've never felt before. The best thing I can hope for is to receive my Verilux HappyLite™ supplemental light system (a.k.a. "my little sunshine") soon. I sure hope it shines some light on me and helps me get a grip on things before it's too late.

All I know is that things have been tense between Keith and me for over a week, and I feel it everywhere in my body—I have pounding headaches, knots in my shoulders, a gross feeling in my stomach, my joints hurt and my lower back burns.

No, this isn't just a mental illness I'm fighting. Stress manifests itself in my body in different ways. It's not healthy and I hate it! The pain has gotten more intense with each passing year. My two saving graces are yoga and Reiki, which help move the negative energy through and out of my body. I always feel more calm and peaceful after class or a treatment.

This situation sucks. It's all up to me. I don't trust anyone. Not with my health. Not with my life. If I weren't well enough to take action and know what I can do to help myself get well again, then I don't think anyone would know what to do. I'd end up back in the mental hospital.

"Who has my back?" I say to Keith. "Where's the net to catch me? I can't do this alone, Keith. I want us to be a team—to be accountable for one another. I can't do this much longer.

"It's really hard and dark, and I'm losing momentum, like a battery running out of juice. Even my voice changes when I'm depressed. I hardly recognize myself.

"I'm lonely and sad, and I don't even feel that anyone can understand my pain. And worse than that, you don't know *what* to do."

I fall into Keith's arms. Crying helps. I let out another round of anger-induced tears.

"I wish I knew how to help, Michelle," he says, rubbing my back.

I sob into his right shoulder. "Just wanting to be around me is nice, especially when everyone else seems to have bailed on me." His sweatshirt absorbs my tears like a towel. "I feel like everyone's abandoned me. Who's around when the going gets tough?"

Silence. My walls are beginning to go up again.

PMS

"Trust in yourself. Your perceptions are often far more accurate than you are willing to believe."
—Claudia Black

"You have got to be kidding me!" I said to my psychiatrist. "I've spent the past 6½ years mastering how to live with bipolar disorder. Now I have PMS symptoms to contend with? Why didn't anyone tell me sooner?"

I mulled over the last six months—six months of me riding on a sheer, emotional roller coaster from hell, not to mention what it was doing to my relationship with Keith. Poor guy. Sometimes I thought he was on the brink of bailing out on me. But, that's not him. I was fairly certain of that. He knew something was wrong and he wanted to be there for me. I don't know how I lucked out in that department. Thank goodness. He's probably the only guy in America willing to stick by my side. Anyone else from my past would have been long gone by now. But not Keith—or Tigger.

"Thank you, God for bringing such a patient, understanding guy into my life" I said, looking up at the ceiling. I wondered how much longer he was going to hang on.

...

Now I have hormonal changes to contend with. I take things personally, and I'm very sensitive to everything that people say. I honestly think that people say and do things to intentionally hurt my feelings. What someone might say to me during my non-PMS time gets a normal human reaction. But when I'm experiencing PMS, everything I hear is ramped up 150 percent. My normal reactions to things get blown way out of proportion. It's almost as if I can't tell reality from fiction (the "monkey mind voices" that go on in my brain.)

It's tricky because my PMS symptoms mimic my bipolar symptoms. It was only when I reached a state of steady emotional balance that I was able to figure out what was going on. My primary doctor promised that after two months I should see a significant change during my PMS time. I'm keeping my fingers crossed. I don't know why, at age 34, my PMS symptoms have decided to flare up out of control every month.

My body then feels like a rocket about to take flight. All it takes is for someone to ignite my brain and "Michelle the monster" takes over for five days prior to my period. Somehow I've learned to live with fluctuations in my body, but I can take no more! I *hate* who I become. I can't even stand to be in my own company, much less anyone else's. That's pretty pathetic. I just know I'm safer if I hang out alone, let the moods pass and then resume my life. I don't have to justify my moods to anyone. Tigger is my one and only saving grace. He and God are the only ones who see and hear it all. I'm a mess. An emotional slimy, tightly wound alarm clock just waiting to be set off.

Who sets me off and when it happens—oh, that's all to chance. I feel like a 2-year-old having temper tantrums—

and yes, I cry and snot drips down my nose and my eyes get swollen and red from crying and I yell because I'M SO DAMN MISERABLE! Why don't men get PMS? Sometimes being a female sucks—and this is one of those times.

I'm just grateful that my doctor addressed it early enough—before World War IV began with those closest to me. Honestly, I don't have enough fight in me to contend with PMS every month. It takes me a week just to recuperate from the symptoms. It's like having an emotional flu and it completely knocks me out—physically and emotionally. I could use some chicken soup for my brain when it happens—if they made it.

Relief was sent my way via an appointment with my psychiatrist. I don't know why the answer didn't come to her sooner, but after describing my symptoms she asked me one question: "Michelle, are you reacting to what people are saying?"

"Well, yes!" I said. "They're a bunch of flaming idiots with no patience or tolerance for mistakes." That's all it took for her to write a referral to see my primary doctor to get the prescription. Well that was a straightforward test. Amen for that.

Later that afternoon at my primary physician's office, the doctor said, "Well, that answers the question. You said this has been happening to you every month for several months in a row now?"

"Yes."

"I'm going to put you on a low-dose estrogen birth control pill. This will help even out your estrogen hormone so you don't have a severe dip each month, which is what's causing you to have such severe PMS symptoms. You should notice a significant change in your mood overall in a couple of months."

"Thank you. But why didn't you tell me sooner?

BIPOLAR NO MORE

...

Waiting at the pharmacy is not one of the highlights of my life, but since I've pretty much ostracized those closest to me, it's up to me to get things done. And that includes picking up my birth control pills. How ironic. I'm not even having sex and I have to take these things. I don't care. As long as they do what they say they do, then I will be a very happy, balanced woman again in a couple of months. Until then…

When I got back to my car, I said a silent prayer: "Please, little birth control pills, do your magic so I can stop turning into monster woman every month." Sitting in my car, I let the engine warm up and my mind began to wander. I can't even stand to be around me and that's pretty bad. I didn't feel like crying. I didn't even feel a sense of relief or a release of weeks of pent-up emotions. It was just something I needed to take care of, like going to the grocery store. No big deal.

The only part that makes me chuckle is the fact I'm not having sex and I'm taking birth control pills. Shoot. I could be the poster person for abstinence at this rate. But, as it turns out, lots of women take birth control pills for their PMS symptoms, so why not join the club, Michelle?

Just as long as I don't gain weight. I couldn't handle that side-effect well. I know medications are getting better about minimizing side-effects. I trust my doctor is right about this one. Constipation and dry mouth I can handle. Gaining weight would do me in. Like driving on the freeway, it would cause me to become increasingly anxious as the numbers creep up the scale, like those on the speedometer.

RELATIONSHIP WITH KEITH

"Listening is a form of accepting."

—Stella Terrill Mann

I don't know *what* or *how* the emphasis on God entered my relationship with Keith. Two and a half months— tah dah! Here I am visiting the word "dating." To me, it means "getting to know someone with the addition of physical contact,"– hugging, holding hands and kissing.

Here I am checking out a religious novel at the bookstore and coming across the book *Kissed Dating Goodbye* by Joshua Harris. I'm soaking up the words. My heart and head want an explanation...and understanding...and ultimately acceptance. I feel an urgent need to share my new knowledge with Keith.

He has no idea what's coming. We always have honest, interesting conversations, but for some reason, when I met him for coffee after yoga last night, he did not look pleased. He appeared tense and serious and uncomfortable. I pick up signals from people quite easily.

Damn. This sucks. I should've just gone home after class I thought to myself.

Great. There's no place to sit. It's hard to have a heart to heart talk when being sandwiched on a couch next to each other. I sip my tea and make small talk. I pray my prior yoga time will keep me calm and relaxed through the evening. I'm conducting a "test" with my anxiety meds, which is my one medication I take as needed. I didn't take one prior to yoga. I wanted to see if being in class and breathing and focusing on the moment would have the same effect—and it did. It took about half-an-hour, but I did calm down. My mind cleared and I followed the soothing, steady sound of the instructor. I felt somewhat hypnotized.

Finally. A table becomes available. Keith's been eyeing it since we came in. Okay, now the *real* conversation can begin. I tell him about dating one person at a time—getting to know them plus having physical contact. It's hard for me to differentiate between "dating" and "girlfriend and boyfriend." Oh! A sudden revelation. Dating is where a lot of courtship occurs. I hope that *never* stops with us. I don't feel anything but sincere caring feelings from him when he gives me two dozen pink roses, cards and other tokens of his affection. *All* of these come from his heart. And the time we spend together is wonderful. I feel safe. My guard is down. He understands me. No one guy I've dated has *ever* cared so much about me. This is *definitely* a welcome change.

I tell him about the book and about my "ah-hah" moment. In order for a relationship to grow and remain strong there *needs* to be a direct link to God. A triangle with God at the top and us at the base. I don't necessarily agree that spending one hour in a building called "church" once a week constitutes a good relationship with God. What about the *rest* of the week? I *choose* to spend time in nature on

RELATIONSHIP

Sundays. This is where *I* find my peace and time with God most beneficial. I feel a strong, direct link where I'm able to have an uninterrupted conversation with him as I walk, as if He's walking by my side. Keith respects this about me.

I'm Catholic and he's Presbyterian, but *more* importantly, we're *both* committed to having God present in our lives. Never before has this conversation arisen about God playing a vital role in *any* of my past relationships with men. But, Keith's different. I know it and God knows it, and I completely believe that He is guiding me along my journey. I'm so thankful that our paths have crossed and now, met.

I was beginning to pull back when I had an inkling that he might be becoming obsessive—calling everyday and wanting to spend so much time alone together. Trigger. Been there. Done that. Isolation from everyone and everything. Hard to breathe.

Warning flag! Oh no, here we go again. Is *that* what the whole conversation of moving from dating to girlfriend/boyfriend is about? Certainty? Security? I've told him *numerous* times that I am probably the most loyal, honest person he'll ever meet. I hope he believes me. I just want for him to be able to relax and enjoy our time together. Sometimes it feels like he's scared I'm going to end our relationship. I have no reason or desire to. I wish he knew that, too.

So, back to the God conversation. He sat across from me, watching me talk. Hoping I was making *some* sort of sense, I told him this "new" importance of God in my life. In *our* lives. If our relationship is to survive in this world we're definitely going to need His guidance. I wanted Keith to understand and agree. We need to be a team. Going into a relationship with God as our guide and having His importance remain as strong for as long as we both shall live. I know *I* can do this. I'm not sure if he views God the same way or understands the importance He has in our lives.

I'm sure we'll have more conversations about this, but I *do* know that before I make the transition to girl-friend/boyfriend that we both agree to be on a faith-based path. This is the *only* way I see this relationship being able to work. I guess that's what they say, "Walk along with Me and know that I am God."

It just amazes me how this new revelation literally popped out of nowhere. But, now's the time. This is the man. I'm committed and I'm listening with open ears, heart and mind. Hopefully Keith is, too. He's the most unique man I've ever met, yet a combination of all the best quali-ties of men from my past—he's a comedian, a therapist, a best friend, the best conversationalist over a cup of coffee and the best vacation partner I've ever known!

IN THE CAR

"Learn to get in touch with the silence within yourself and know that everything in this life has a purpose."
—Elisabeth Kübler-Ross

I've found the best time to discuss things with Keith is in the car, where I find it both safe and productive. We both have to be in the car going to the same destination, so we might as well make the most of it, turn off the radio and listen to each other's concerns, gripes, disappointments or problems. And as we head toward our destination, we know we have "X" amount of time to talk about a subject, so we adjust accordingly and finish the conversation before exiting the car.

When did we start doing this? I don't remember. Keith is very easy to talk to, and it amazes me that, although he's the introvert in our relationship, he does most of the talking. And he's a very interesting conversationalist. Sometimes I'd honestly rather talk to him than some of my girlfriends. He has depth and a variety of interests (and I don't even mind listening to him carry on about golf.) I can tell he's passionate about it and truth be told, it's nice seeing him get excited about something.

After the holidays, we drove to Santa Fe, New Mexico,

to visit some of his family (some of his family equals 20-plus people, whereas all of my family equals 11 people).

I was incredibly peeved that he didn't remember our one-year anniversary. Funny thing, though, he remembers all of our important dates and I don't—not that I don't want to, but it's nice he cares so much and wants to remember them. How he managed to forget our one-year anniversary, I don't know, but I do recall how I felt—slighted, unimportant. One year! That's a huge deal in my book, especially because this is the first relationship I've had in over six years.

I mean, come on people. How about some flowers— delivered by a singing telegram would have been a nice touch—how about writing me a poem or a love letter, or take me on a road trip. I'm not asking for the world. I just want to feel special for one day—to feel loved and appreciated and acknowledged. My feelings, by the way, have been constant throughout our relationship. It just hurt more on our anniversary day because IT WAS OUR ANNIVERSARY DAY. Make it special, for heaven's sake. I pray that next year will be better.

We had one hour in the car to discuss my displeasure. He apologized almost every 15 minutes, and he gave me a very thoughtful card and photo frame to make peace. It worked. I can't stay mad at him. I love him. I know eventually I'm going to screw up, or forget something, and it'll be his turn to forgive me. I think that's one of my big lessons to learn: how to forgive, forget and move on.

We had a lovely time at the party, and driving home was much more relaxed. We listened to Delilah—I've converted him to her weekly evening dedication program—and held hands (the car has an automatic transmission). We didn't have much to say to each other, just recapped the events of the evening.

It was great meeting more of his family, and I really had an enjoyable time. He has a good, loving family. He's lucky. I am, too. It's rare. How we found each other in this big ol' planet I don't know.

Actually, I do know. God had a hand in it. It just took time and patience.

...

It's been two days since the accident. I can't get it out of my mind. I wasn't even involved in it, thank goodness.

"Hey Keith, wanna' go grab some dinner? I brought the Entertainer book."

"Sure. Anything but Mexican, right? How about this pizza place?" he replied.

"Sounds good. Let's go. I'm starving," I said.

His car had been acting up recently, so I drove. Turning on our favorite radio station to listen to Delilah, I pulled out of his driveway and headed east.

We had spent the afternoon together and amazingly still had things to talk about. That's one of the things I like about Keith. We can have a conversation about anything. He's easy to talk to as well as a good listener.

"What in the world?" I said as I turned at the light and immediately saw all the police car bubble lights up ahead. My heart began to speed up. I hate seeing accidents and this one was fresh.

"Don't look, Michelle. Don't look. Turn the other way. Focus straight ahead," I told myself verbally as we approached the bright lights of a multitude of cop cars. I focused on gripping the steering wheel and watching the way the light was hitting my nail polish causing it to shimmer in the sunlight. "I've got to remain in control. Get a grip, Michelle" I told myself mentally.

163

But, being the curious person that I am, I looked. And I regret it. Immensely. If a picture is worth a thousand words, then I should have no trouble meeting the word count for this chapter.

What I saw was absolutely horrific. I can't even stand to watch horror movies on TV. And this was real life and I was shaken to the core. I don't even know how I managed to drive us to the restaurant. I was shaking like a diabetic needing insulin immediately.

Writing about this will hopefully help me heal. But the painful memory is so new I don't know how I'll react. There was a car and a motorcycle. As we were approaching the accident I looked over my left shoulder and just for a brief moment was able to capture everything I needed to put all the puzzle pieces together.

There was a motorcycle on its side and not far behind it was a thick off-white colored sheet covering a long, big lump in the middle of the road.

"I think I'm going to throw up, Keith." I felt nauseous and shaky. My reaction happened so fast. I didn't know the people who were involved in the accident. My overactive, vivid imagination filled in the blanks of what might be lying beneath the sheet. Thank goodness they had covered the body in time; otherwise, I think I would have gotten physically ill right there on the spot.

"Keith, promise me you'll never ride a motorcycle," I asked him in a shaky voice.

"I promise, Michelle," he replied as he reached for my hand and squeezed it tight to reassure me.

There was a four door car up the road a ways. I didn't see people in it. I didn't see people involved in the accident anywhere. Were they all dead? Was it a hit and run? There were too many questions for me to comprehend.

I thought getting some food in my stomach might help.

I ate some at the restaurant. Our moods had definitely sub-
dued after witnessing the accident. Damn, why did we have
to witness that accident? We had a pleasant afternoon and
then *bam* something comes along so out of the blue that
neither of us knows what to do with it.

"I can't drive back to your house the usual way. Is there
an alternate route I can take?" I asked him.

"Yeah, not a problem. We can go the back way," he
said.

I wasn't sure if the accident scene had been cleaned up
yet and I certainly was not up to driving over where it had
occurred. It was too fresh in my mind. How long was this
going to take me to recover from?

We went back to his place and watched TV for awhile.
I still couldn't get my mind off of the accident. I had a
strong urge to go home. I needed to be around a lot of security and comforting and familiarity and these included my
home, Tigger, my parents and my room.

Driving home I decided to travel the route past where
the accident occurred. By this time, several hours had
passed and it was as if nothing has happened. But my body
and mind knew otherwise.

"I need you to "escort" me home, Keith," I asked him
in his front yard.

"Sure. I'll wait for your call," he said.

I got in my car and before I reached the end of his street
I had dialed his phone number. A method I came up with to
make sure I made it home okay, I would dial his number
and put it on speaker phone on the front passenger's seat so
he could keep me company and make sure I made it home
okay.

"Okay Keith, I really need for you to talk to me here.
I'm approaching the accident site and I'm feeling nervous.
Keith, talk to me."

There was silence. Why isn't he talking to me? Is something wrong with my phone? Can you hear me? I said.

"Yes, I can hear you, Michelle."

"I really need your help here getting past these next few lights," I said semi-panicked.

"I don't know what to say," he said.

Great. A time when I need him the most and...keep it together, Michelle. You can do this. You've driven this route a lot. It's no big deal, just breathe, I told myself. I grabbed the steering wheel even tighter and focused like a race car driver with blinders on.

One light, two lights and three lights. Okay, and exhale. It's okay, Michelle. Breathe, I told myself.

The rest of the ride was uncomfortable. I was begging him for conversation—anything. It was like me learning to drive stick shift, jerky and awkward and frustrating.

This isn't like us. What happened to the great conversations we had earlier that day? Did he only have so much conversation material in him and then he ran dry? Where are you, Keith? I need you. I can't go through this alone. You saw just as much as I did of that accident. Please don't leave me to go through this alone. I felt desperately sad.

I couldn't cry or get mad. I was stuck—no, I was in shock.

...

It wasn't until 24 hours had passed that my emotions rose to the surface. It happened fast and my parents were the ones who received the shocking news of what I'd experienced the evening before. It's no wonder I can't watch the evening news or read the daily newspaper. The amount and severity of bad news that plasters the media is too much for me to handle.

IN THE CAR

My mom was watching TV and I could barely muster out, "Would you mind turning off the TV, I need to talk to you."

As soon as she hit the power button my tears poured out and with it came the loss and frustration from the accident and from Keith. Everything was wrapped up like in a messy burrito and everything came out in wracking sobs.

"That must be really hard, what you're going through and trying to process it," my dad said as he sat next to me and rubbed my back like a young child. It was soothing and was what I could have used from Keith the night before. But being in shock I didn't know what I needed the previous night.

Keith had held me in his arms while we watched TV for awhile to try and distract ourselves. "Men in Black" was not my first choice, but there wasn't a whole lot else on that was relatively interesting. I remember that the slime in the movie reminded me of blood and I covered my eyes during most of it. My shaken up self could've really used a good comedy movie—or "Will and Grace" reruns.

I just wracked out in uncontrollable sobs what I'd seen. I did throw up the night before, but it was from extreme menstrual cramps not the image of the dead person covered by a sheet.

"I don't know if I'll ever be able to drive down that street again where the accident occurred." Driving over where the dead body was made me squirm thinking of it.

"It could take some time, Michelle. Maybe it's a good idea to talk to your therapist about this. Maybe she can help you process it so it doesn't continue to haunt you," said my dad.

"That's a good idea. I see her on Wednesday. Until then I'm just going to try and distract myself."

...

It wasn't until later Sunday evening when I was in my room that it hit me. Why was I feeling nauseous and having an unsettling feeling? It went beyond seeing the motorcycle accident—it went back to Warren and after I was diagnosed.

How I got the two incidents to tie together, I do not know. But it hit me like an Oprah "ah hah moment." For several years after I was diagnosed I could not bring myself to drive past Warren's house. He lived on the same street as me and I purposely found an alternate route to take when I had to travel in his direction to run errands, visit my parents and whatever else caused me to travel in his direction.

I remember initially getting very anxious whenever I'd get in my car and think about passing by his house. I didn't want anything to do with him anymore. He had ruined my life enough, the disgusting pig. I wanted to clear my conscience of him as much and as quickly as possible.

I never realized how long it can take to get over a tragic event. For me, it lingered in my brain for five years. I would have flashbacks of the time we spent together and unfortunately the times he took advantage of me inevitably surfaced as well.

Every so often throughout the five year period that followed my diagnosis I would "test" myself and see how I reacted when I drove by his house. I think I somehow knew that eventually I would be healed from his memories and be able to drive by his house and be just fine with it.

Over time, it got easier and his memory continued to lessen. I would sing along to the radio and look away when I approached his house. Little by little it got easier to drive past his house. My anxiety lessoned.

I'm proud to say that the past two years have been fine. I drive by his house and think nothing. It's a house and our encounter happened such a long time ago it seems like another lifetime to me. He has no hold on me or my memories. He was part of my past life and that's where he's remaining. I have complete faith that his karma will take care of things.

So, how does this relate to the motorcycle accident? Well, I believe that over time, I'm not sure how long it will take for my mind to heal from seeing what I did, but I trust that at some point in time I'll be able to drive down that road again and be fine with it. The memory of it will lessen over time and eventually I believe that I won't think about the accident at all. I'm just very thankful that I didn't know the people involved. Seeing it was tragic enough for my sensitive self.

The accident happened on the road to the church I attend. For now, I'll drive around the back way. Yes, church is *that* important to me. And it's been a long time since I found a church that I feel is a good fit for my needs. I look forward to it each week. And if driving an alternate route is what it takes, then so be it. It's only a temporary thing, and I know, that like with Warren, I'll be able to put the motorcycle accident behind me and focus on my destination—church.

WHAT'S GOD SAYING?

"Desire, ask, believe, receive."

—Stella Terrill Mann

No amount of chocolate eating could pacify the emotional pain I'm in right now. Last night was horrible—as well as the definitive answer to my prayer.

While looking at my reflection in the mirror this morning I could barely audibly make it through my daily morning prayer:

I have to live with myself and so
I want to be fit for myself to know
I want to be able as days go by
Always to look myself straight in the eye
I don't want to stand with the setting sun
And hate myself for the things I've done

"Things I've done? Oh Lord. This is just about the most difficult thing I've *ever* gone through. God, where did my relationship with Keith go wrong?"

I thought I had my answer a couple of weeks ago after attending a private spiritual retreat. It was exactly what my soul needed. Time away to reflect on the strengths of our relationship, things I thought we needed to work on and ultimately, to decide if Keith was the man I wanted to move forward with in our relationship, or if I wanted to be alone or with someone else. (There currently is no "someone else.")

I promised myself a very long time ago that I would never settle—for anything. Whether that's a mediocre relationship or an okay job so I can pay the bills. It's not me. Never has been. Never will be. I am a very independent, strong willed woman and I want the best in life. I'm definitely willing to work for it and to make sacrifices along the way.

The answer of whether to stay with Keith or move on became very clear to me during my retreat. I felt God's closeness, that He was protecting me and that yes, staying with Keith was the right thing to do. I never doubt God. I just trust Him that He is guiding me and is presenting things into my life out of love.

Before I returned home from my retreat, I knew for certain the next step I needed to take. I registered us for an evening couple's retreat—married and unmarried were welcome. When I mentioned it to Keith several weeks prior, he seemed interested. I thought this would put us on the right path to pursuing a faith-based relationship overseen by God. For the 15 months I've dated Keith, he's always been open to doing things that I bring to our relationship. He hasn't turned down a single activity. It amazes me and I appreciate his openness. Some of the things—whether it's painting pottery, country dance lessons or taking road trips, he's said "yes" to all of these things and more. I'm very thankful he has an open mind and is open to new adventures with me.

But sitting in class last night, I looked around and some of the couples were either holding hands, smiling lovingly at each other or sharing some little story that was just between them. It was sweet. I could see the love they shared and I wondered, where's ours?

The priest went over the five ingredients to a happy marriage. This was to be a preparatory ground for Keith and my relationship. My taking a relationship break was a good opportunity for us both to regroup. I was hoping that when we met again a week and half later that things would change—for the better. I told Keith that I'd prayed about our relationship and it felt like we were drifting apart. And I knew why. God wasn't in it. "There are three things I'd like for us to do in order for our relationship to move forward—attend the evening for couples, start going to church and going to visit your brother and his family this summer."

I felt confident sharing these things with him. It felt the timing was right and as I had hoped, Keith was open and willing to participate. "Thank you, God, for using me as a vessel to help reach Keith. I really want our relationship to work. I pray that you please continue to guide us on the right path."

Driving home after the evening relationship session I was looking forward to sharing with Keith some of my thoughts. I felt like I'd been filled with hope. One thing I love about our relationship is our conversations. We've had some great, meaningful discussions and I become closer to him because of them. Tonight however, was not the case. I could feel his defenses going up, higher and higher. "Why? I'm not going to bite your head off? You haven't acted this way in the past. What's changed?" I thought to myself. I asked lots of questions, trying to get him to open up. "Come on Keith, I know you're in there somewhere. Just talk to me. If we don't have communication, then we don't have anything" I say to myself.

I look at him out of the corner of my eye. His lips are

tight. He looks like he's sitting in a straight jacket. He's focused on something, but I don't know what. I'm pretty good at picking up on people's nonverbal communication and he's communicating pretty well that he does not want to be there. Whether "there" means partaking in our conversation, riding in my car or something else about the evening, I do not know. This was supposed to be a *fun* evening. A chance for us to start over and slowly feel God's presence in our lives. I'm at the starting line, revving my engine waiting for you to show up. I don't want to race you; I want to ride along side you.

I thought we were a team, I tell him as I glance over to hopefully get eye contact with him. I feel like you're pulling away, like you're done trying. You've gone through the whole "wooing" phase of trying to impress me, get my attention and earn my love. Yes, you've done all of those things, but they never end. Not in my mind anyway. It feels like "couch potato" city and you've run out of methods to show your continued love for me, energy that needs to keep being poured into the pitcher to keep it alive by *both* of us. My worst fear—you've done what you had to do to "win me over." You've passed the class with flying colors, done everything by the book and now you think "Michelle is mine."

The only thing is that I'm not yours to have. God brought us together for very special reasons. I feel myself moving forward with my life and I sense your negativity and complacency grow each day. I need to be with someone who can make me laugh. Someone who treats me like the special woman that I am—not a queen, but doing little things backed up with love, like an occasional congratulatory card or flowers or going out and doing things. Even holding my hand while we take a walk is nice. I will *never* settle, Keith. I thought you were the one.

WHAT'S GOD SAYING?

I'm doubting God and I'm doubting myself. Something I rarely do. I thought God gave me the go ahead sign with our relationship, but now I'm having second thoughts. I do know one thing though; I'm choosing not to move forward with the state our relationship is in. We're sinking and I can't swim. Life's too short. I've been through seven years of emotional and mental pain, it's time for me to have some fun. I thought the person I'd be sharing this joy with was you.

The dreaded "f" word surfaces to my lips. I don't want to cut you out of my life forever. The past 15 months we've shared I wouldn't trade for anything. But, I feel we're growing apart and I *need* to be with someone who treats me special. I need it like I need *air.* But also, I deserve it. I feel you slipping away, slipping into your comfort zone and forgetting what we used to have. I want us to be friends. For now anyway, until I can figure out what I need in a relationship. I hope that with time will come understanding, for both of us. I love you, Keith.

Delilah must have known what was on my heart the evening this conversation occurred. Getting ready for bed, I turned on my radio and moved the mountain of pillows from my bed to the floor. The timing couldn't have been any more perfect. I took in a breath, then turned to look at the stereo. How could she know the song I was thinking about? Michael Bublé began to sing "Lost." I immediately folded myself up on the floor next to my bed, let my hair drape all around me, like a curtain, and I just sobbed as I listened to this sad, beautiful song.

"Please, help me God, I plead out loud through wracking sobs. I'm not strong enough to handle this. I can't even breathe. What have I done? Did I just go and scare off the greatest guy I've even dated? Great Michelle, way to go. Run another one away so you won't get hurt. What's wrong with me? Why can't I make a relationship work?"

Slowly, Michael's voice blended into my thoughts.

I thought you were the one. I trusted you.

I had hope. I had faith in God that He brought us together. I chose to ignore our challenges, living only for happy times.

I never thought it would end this way. Saying good-bye is so very hard to do, but it's what I must do. God's calling me in a different direction now. Good-bye, Keith.

NAMI- "IN OUR OWN VOICE"

"Take a risk a day—one small or bold stroke that will make you feel great once you have done it."
—Susan Jeffers

It's now been four years that I've been giving "In Our Own Voice" (IOOV) presentations to inpatients at several local psychiatric hospitals, which I consider to be the ultimate blessing of having bipolar disorder. I feel it's a gift from God to give hope to others who have recently been diagnosed. He gives me the strength and courage and the words to say. Each time I do a presentation, my goal is that I reach one person in the audience. Being able to connect with the audience and address questions and concerns makes me feel that I'm making a difference—that something I say will ring true for them and will prevent them from having to go through what I did when I was first diagnosed seven years ago.

Unfortunately, IOOV didn't exist in Albuquerque when I was first hospitalized. Consequently, when I was discharged as a newly diagnosed mentally-ill patient, I had only my doctor and my parents to rely on for answering my endless questions. But to no avail– it just wasn't enough. It was like dousing a sunburned person with aloe, waiting for the burning to stop and the redness to disappear—only my burning was taking place on the inside and nothing, not words or medication, seemed to soothe it.

I'll never forget those first couple of horrific years with my condition. I wouldn't wish that kind of emotional pain on anyone. I think that's the main reason why I present. It helps me heal. And it keeps me humble. With each passing year, I feel that helping others helps me become a whole person again. Although I'll never be the woman I was before I was diagnosed, I am much stronger, both mentally and emotionally. The IOOV presentations give inpatients an opportunity to see what it's like to be mentally well. That you can have a life after being diagnosed and it's definitely possible to have a positive recovery.

I'm very thankful I'm able to do something constructive with my illness. Both giving presentations and writing my book are wonderful, creative outlets for me. I feel a strong connection with others when I speak and write about my brain disorder.

In college, I never considered myself to be a great public speaker. As a matter of fact, I frequently froze when I went to the front of the class to deliver a presentation for one of my marketing classes. Looking around the classroom at some 200-plus people I couldn't breathe. I got anxious. My mind went blank and I thought I was going to pass out. But I didn't. I thought I was thoroughly prepared with my research done and notes in hand. My mouth went dry and I said "um" a million times. I felt like I was sinking in quicksand and everyone in the room was watching me go deeper and deeper. It was embarrassing and I just wanted to hide.

Oh, dear God, I would think. Please help me make it

IOOV

through this presentation. I know the material. I know I can do this. Please help me say the right thing:

...

"Hi. My name's Michelle. I'm here on behalf of the National Alliance on Mental Illness (NAMI) to talk to you about a program called "In Our Own Voice" (IOOV).

"There are five sections to the presentation. They are Dark Days, Acceptance, Treatment, Coping Skills and Successes, Hopes and Dreams. After each section there will be time for questions and discussion.

Just a little bit about myself. I'm 34 years old. I live at home with my parents and my dog, Tigger. I enjoy clogging, camping, watching comedy movies, traveling and scrapbooking. I've been giving IOOV presentations for four years to inpatients at several local psychiatric hospitals, the local university, to nursing students and at churches.

"Presenting here at the UNM Mental Health Center is the newest outreach for IOOV. This hospital is 'home' to me. This is where I was first diagnosed and hospitalized in May 2001. I was in this very ward."

It doesn't feel weird or uncomfortable to me walking down the hallway where I was initially escorted by two police officers on May 24, 2001. I've never been one who likes going to hospitals, but this one is only two floors so I don't feel the least bit anxious.

I didn't know what to expect when I gave my first several presentations at the Mental Health Center. I retraced my steps to the desk where I was given a pee cup, then taken into the time-out room for my Adavan shot, given a dinner tray and shown to my room. I was definitely seeing things through a filter when I was admitted. The memories are all there for me to relive, but they don't seem as raw and *Cops*-like now. It's amazing what time—and medications can do.

I realize we're all in this together—the inpatients and me—and this is what keeps it real for me. It means that, yes, I really do have this illness, and I had better continue taking good care of myself because there's a fine line between staying well and becoming ill again. I could end up as an inpatient here again. The mere thought of that makes me shutter. I'll do anything to keep from coming back here. Fortunately, I'm doing so well that I can't fathom that ever occurring. I pray every day that God continues to watch over me and helps me stay well.

Giving these presentations is very humbling and a regular reminder of how far I've come in my own recovery process. Sometimes it amazes me just how far I have come. I know it's all possible because of my faith in God, my treatment team—psychiatrist, nurse and therapist, supportive parents—as well as faithfully taking my medications each day, living in my environment, monitoring my stress, walking my dog daily for exercise and the positive local and long-distance friendships.

I sometimes wonder if the absence of what I have is what prevents those with a mental illness from reaching a high level of recovery—meaning being able to work, having relationships and feeling fulfilled. I know that everyone's needs are different, but shouldn't there be an equation or formula for a successful recovery? I wonder sometimes why I'm able to live such a full, happy life while living with this illness and yet others struggle with the most basic of needs. Is it our illness—or something else?

I would love to do research and find out answers to this and other questions that I have been pondering for several years. I feel that I've reached the highest possible point in my recovery process without a "cure." I feel like a regular,

normal person living my life just like everyone else.
I'm managing my illness daily, yet it's not at the forefront of my mind. My bipolar disorder is a part of me—not
all of me. I no longer let it define me or hold me back. I
feel more comfortable taking risks. I feel myself evolving
more and more into the woman I want to be with each passing day. My illness has allowed me the opportunity to examine my life, something I don't think would have
happened otherwise.

"I was a successful college graduate with a marketing
degree who worked in advertising for five years before
having my acute manic breakthrough that ended up with
me here at the Mental Health Center. It was an absolute
whirlwind experience and I found myself paralyzed with
the severity and intensity of it all. My Dark Days began after I was diagnosed and lasted for about two years. I lost
everything—overnight. My job, home, boyfriend, friends
and dignity were gone, faster than I could swallow.

"I was hospitalized for seven days until I was stable on
my medications and my doctor released me. I had nowhere
to go, so I had to move back home and live with my parents.
Fortunately, my room was still my room, almost like they
were expecting me to live with them again at some point.
Without their hospitality I would have been out on the
streets. That thought makes me shudder. I feel very blessed
at my parents' willingness to take me back in, like a bird
with an injury, to help nurse me back to health."

I don't know what it was like from their viewpoint having to take care of my every need. We never talk about my
Dark Days. I think it's still very raw for them. To see their
successful, independent daughter crash and have to return
home and start over—honestly—who would want that for
their child? I do know they prayed a lot and cried. And they
always made sure I was taken care of and that I had every-

thing I needed, physically and mentally.

I remember my mom going with me to every psychiatrist appointment I had for the first year until I was comfortable and strong enough to go on my own. She and my dad also came to weekly DBSA meetings with me for several months to make sure I was comfortable. It kind of reminded me of when they took me to kindergarten as a young child. Shaky and on the verge of tears, they would stay with me until I had met some friends and was having a good time. Only then would they go to work.

They instinctively knew I needed help and never complained about having to leave work early to take me to a doctor's appointment or go to a DBSA meeting after having been at work all day. Having their support at this very beginning stage was crucial and I don't think I'd be where I am today if it weren't for their endless help.

Because of my instability, for awhile my dad made special trips to the pharmacy each month to get my medications. My low co-pays for my medications were a direct result of him helping me fill out financial-aid paperwork, which also made my doctor visits affordable. It's expensive to be sick and scary as hell at what it costs for doctor visits and medications. Seeing those prices was enough to make me depressed.

My mom and dad helped me fill out the necessary paperwork and went with me to my financial aid appointments where they could explain the situation on my behalf. I could hardly think straight, much less talk clearly to people where I'd make sense. Everything in my brain felt all garbled, and they helped put things in order and make sense.

Short of helping me use the bathroom, my parents did everything for me for a solid two years. I'm sure it was exhausting. But like most parents, I'm sure they were hoping I would come around. They never tried to hurry my recovery process. I'd suffered a blow to the brain and it was going to take time to heal. They had an incredible amount of patience during this time.

After about six months it felt like my medications were beginning to take effect. I couldn't work, so I just sat at my parents' home in a chair and cried—for hours on end. I was numb. I didn't know what to think. It felt like not only was my brain broken, but that I was broken, too. I'd never cried so long and so hard. I cried down to my very soul, feeling that no one could understand me. It felt like my life was over—until something happened.

•••

"The second section of the IOOV presentation is called Acceptance. A good couple of years passed by before I reached this stage. And what helped, you might ask? Seeing a list of support groups on the back of my psychiatrist's door during one of my appointments, I noticed there was a group called the Depression and Bipolar Support Alliance (DBSA).

"My heart skipped a beat. You mean there's help for people who have a mental illness? I was intrigued. I asked my mom to go to the first several meetings with me. I'd never gone to a support group before and it was reassuring to have her sit next to me.

"I didn't say anything beyond introductions. I didn't want anyone to know my story. Not yet. It was too fresh and too real. I just sat and listened while the others shared. I could relate to what some of them were sharing and I returned week after week."

Little by little I began to accept my illness. My illness was very much most of me at that beginning stage. I felt like a walking illness—one that everyone could see when they looked at me. Yep, she's got bipolar written all over her. I was ashamed to look at people and for the most part this is what kept me at home for two years. I don't know why, but I thought there was a certain look a bipolar person had. Crazy, but true. Me and my overactive imagination. Sometimes it was *not* helpful.

While beginning to accept my illness, I took my medications faithfully each day, went to my psychiatrist appointments, DBSA meetings, yoga and walked my dog each day. This was my world for the better part of two years. Small and simple and quiet. Exactly what I needed to begin to heal.

My parents also were affected by my illness. They attended a twelve-week "Family to Family" class sponsored by the National Alliance on Mental Illness (NAMI) a year after my diagnosis. It was very helpful for them to help understand me and my needs, as well as to give them a safe place to share their feelings. They also became quite active in local NAMI events, especially the annual fundraising NAMIWalks.

Probably the biggest change during my acceptance stage was acknowledging my limitations. Prior to my diagnosis I had a lot more energy and could go the better part of a day before feeling the effects of exhaustion. Something changed, I'm not sure exactly what, but I was no longer able to keep going at the same pace or do the same amount of activities after my diagnosis.

I would get mentally exhausted easily, like a runner continuously trying to catch her breath. I was finding myself able to do things only for short spurts of time, like 30 minutes, and then needing to rest. It was incredibly frustrating and I often pushed myself to mental exhaustion. Like learning to drive stick shift and applying too much gas before letting up on the clutch, I had to relearn my inner timing and it was going to be tough.

It was at that stage that I created daily activity cards— simple 3 x 5 index cards on colored paper. There's one for each day of the week—Monday through Friday. An example of one of these cards: Thursday's activities. Below that I list four activities that I need to accomplish that day. Why four? Because this allows me the time and energy to get everything done. Each activity takes approximately one hour to complete. I leave enough time and space for one or two extra activities as things come up, like having lunch with a friend or a dental appointment. Then I know that I'll have both the time *and* the energy for these extra activities. Thursday's card includes walking Tigger, writing, vacuuming the house and helping with dinner.

Fridays are the exception. There's no work, only play on Fridays. For example, I'll go to a museum, visit a friend, go to lunch, visit a bookstore or watch a movie. I really like my three-day weekends—my personal reward for a week of good work.

Anyone can use these cards. I know they're incredibly beneficial for me. They help keep me on track and focused for the day. They also help diminish my anxiety level, which is especially high when I wake up in the morning. Seeing these cards on my desk helps me to breathe, focus and they reassure me that I can get things done.

I've used the cards for five years and, as a positive result, have needed to rely less on my anxiety medication. I now take it only as needed because I'm able to mentally reduce my anxiety by seeing what needs to get done. The pattern of using these reassuring cards for several years calms me down.

"The third section of my presentation is called Treatment, which I consider to be like the layers of lasagna. It includes my medications, which often leave me with dry mouth. My parents, doctors and friends are the second layer.

Yoga, journaling, and walking Tigger are layers three through five. Giving IOOV presentations is healing for me and is layer six. Dancing, both clogging and country, is layer seven. And having positive people in my life and things to look forward to are the remaining eighth and ninth layers.

"These are things that I deem important in my life. Everyone's treatment plan is going to look different. It took me time and introspection to arrive at the things that comprise my treatment plan. Each is equally important and, over time, I may add more lasagna layers. But, for now, these are the things that allow me to stay well—on all levels, physically, mentally, emotionally and spiritually. The important thing is to have balance: some work and some play. Some alone time and some time with people, doctors and medication and even some time in your home environment."

I talk in detail about coping in the book's next section. In my presentation to the inpatients I share that I no longer watch the evening news or read the newspaper. Reading and seeing the overly prevalent negative things cause me anxiety and excessive worrying. I told my parents if there's good news, please share it with me. Otherwise, I can't handle hearing about all the negative things going on in the city or the world. It's too much for me to handle and really throws me off balance. I become depressed and withdrawn and find myself crying over things I cannot control. I choose to focus on the positive things in life.

I also have a morning prayer session that helps me handle my anxiety I experience when I first wake up and which lasts for several hours. I have a bubbling fountain I listen to and I read from an inspirational Bible book, which helps get me focused for the day and connect with God. I've been doing this for a couple of years and it really does make a difference. Whatever's on my mind, I talk to God. I know He's there to help me and guide me on my life's journey. I spend about 15 minutes doing this. Then I recite a public domain poem I bought from a calligrapher at an arts and crafts fair. She abridged it from one titled "Myself" by Edgar Guest:

I have to live with myself and so
I want to be fit for myself to know,
I want to be able, as the days go by,
Always to look myself straight in the eye;
I don't want to stand with the setting sun,
And hate myself for the things I've done.
I want to go out with my head erect,
I want to deserve everyone's respect;
For here in the struggle for fame and self
I want to be able to like myself.
I don't want to look at myself and know
I'm a cheat, a liar and an empty show.
I never can hide myself from me;
I see what others may never see;
I know what others may never know,
I never can fool myself and so,
Whatever happens, I want to be
Self-respecting and conscience free.

I've learned to listen to myself and, with practice and time, I can usually tell what I need. It really is the ultimate in self-care. It's like grown-up Michelle taking care of inner-child Michelle. I try to be kind to myself and not beat up myself mentally because I can't keep up with everyone else, or because my needs are different from others. I just know that whatever activity I choose to participate in will have a consequence. I know I'll have to pay—energy-wise.

It's been this way for years and I just accept it and go with it. I'm not ashamed or embarrassed. I'm thankful that I can take such good care of myself.

"The final section of my IOOV presentation is called Successes, Hopes and Dreams. I'm proud to say that I've been stable on my medications for five years. I feel I have a good balanced life between work and play. I take really good care of myself and this actually spills over into my relationships with others. My relationships are very important to me and I spend quality time nurturing them and making them as strong as possible. To build trust, I strive for honesty, good communication and laughter. The people who are in my life since I've been diagnosed are now all new relationships. They are good people who have my best interest at heart and most importantly, they like me for *me*.

"I like to end my presentation with a quote from Henry David Thoreau. 'Go confidently in the direction of your dreams. Live the life you've imagined.' May this presentation give you hope that you too can achieve a full recovery, no matter what stage you're at in your recovery process."

JURY DUTY

"The Universe will reward you for taking risks on its behalf."
—Shakti Gawain

Me? Jury duty? Now, there are two words I thought I'd never see side-by-side in my lifetime. Nonetheless, it's true. I was selected to spend two weeks of my life at the District Court in downtown Albuquerque.

I hadn't been downtown since I worked for the radio station where I sold airtime. Actually, District Court is right across the street from that station's buildings. Of the two, I'm glad to be going to serve jury duty. There's purpose and a time frame. And, this is just part of my life—not the rest of it.

I must admit, when I received my jury summons in the mail, I was not thrilled at all. My schedule was just fine. Things were moving along smoothly and then—bam! Congratulations, the letter implied, your life will now officially be put on hold so you can help us determine the good versus bad persons in previously selected cases. (It was presented more formally in the letter, but that was how I interpreted it.)

189

Man, you've got to be kidding me, I said to myself. I don't wanna' do this. It said on the back of the form, under Request for Excuse, "If you have an extreme mental, physical or financial hardship, please fill out the appropriate forms. The Court will review them and you'll be notified of a decision." Perfect. My ticket to freedom. Thank you, mental illness.

I left a voicemail for my psychiatrist so she could write me a note to be excused. I honestly did not feel emotionally stable enough to sit and listen for extended periods of time and make really important decisions determining if someone is innocent or guilty. Now, that's stressful. What if I made the wrong decision? I thought. I'm almost sure the court system is reserved for those who are "normal" people. Honestly, there are days when I can't decide what pair of socks to wear. Do other people struggle with this as well? Is it due to the lighting or just a general lack of decision-making abilities?

I also wondered if I would want someone with a mental illness making a decision about *my* future if I were on trial. I guess it would depend on that person's mental and emotional stability at the time of the trial. I honestly felt that once the judge began sharing information with us about the trial that I just might break down crying.

As jurors, we're not allowed to discuss the case before us, and I'm certain that goes for writing about it, as well. I felt very much engulfed in a trial cocoon. It was probably a good thing that I wasn't selected for the trial. I'm almost certain that I would have broken down and cried in the jury box or in deliberations. Are jurors allowed to cry? I don't watch a lot of court TV shows, but the ones I have seen have no crying. I most definitely could not maintain a poker face. I'm much too emotional a person and I think my illness has brought out my emotions more—not a bad thing, but something that I definitely notice.

Suppressing my emotions is like suffocating myself. I find I feel much better the sooner I can release my emotions, whatever they might be. Like letting the air out of a balloon, it may be ugly, but at least I can return to being balanced after I do so. I think if I were selected to serve on a jury I'd be a walking emotional time bomb just waiting to explode. Lashing out comments and crying probably isn't allowed during a trial, but it would make the case a bit more interesting. That's for sure!

I honestly didn't know if I'd have difficulty staying awake, avoiding fidgeting in my seat or even focusing for long periods of time. I thought I was doing the judicial system a favor. My doctor saw otherwise. She did not write me an excuse and my nurse informed me during my next appointment that both my doctor and therapist thought I was perfectly capable of going to jury duty.

I was pissed. "You people are supposed to be part of my treatment team," I said, "meaning that you work with me. You're not working with me here. I have a simple request and I can't believe you're not going to help me out."

"Michelle," my therapist said, "we think you are perfectly capable of going to jury duty. Don't sell yourself short. You're more well than you think you are."

"Yeah, because I take really good care of myself. Who knows what two weeks of jury duty's going to do to my mental status? Guess I'm going to find out because I'm going to jury duty. Lucky me."

Yeah, I felt about as lucky as a shiny penny that had been pooped on by a dog with diarrhea. I stalked out of my therapist's office, fuming. I can't believe those people. Crap. Two weeks.

I told my parents about the jury duty that night. They seemed glad I was going. They actually agreed with my doctor that I am doing really well.

All righty then, I thought. Let's see what will put Michelle over the top. It felt like everyone was against me. They wanted to see how far they could push me before I broke and ended up back at the Mental Health Center. Well, if I did, it would be their own damn fault and I'd make sure that they'd really regret their decision.

Hah! Fooled you. Not as strong as I seem, I told myself.

...

In the end, the joke was on me. Or was it reality was on me? I was fine. From day one. I packed my lunch the night before, something I hadn't done since grade school. I took my clothes out that I was going to wear the next day and off to bed I went.

My alarm was set for 6:00 AM. Oh geez, when was the last time I woke up at that ungodly hour? Zero hour for band? It's still dark outside. Need caffeine. Lots of caffeine. My usual 7:30 AM gentle wakeup would be in hiatus for a couple of weeks. I'd better get used to this.

What is with the traffic? It was 20 minutes of moderate traffic. Fortunately, parking was close by and was paid for. I am so fortunate that the "commute" to my home office is all of 10 feet from my bedroom. I definitely do not miss the commute thing.

With a 9:15 AM report time, I was half an hour early. I can't stand being late. Besides, I didn't know exactly where I was going. I wanted ample time to scope things out. Good thing for instincts. I wasn't the only one summoned to appear for jury duty that morning in February. There was a line out to the street. There must have been about 100 people in front of me. No way! How many cases are going on today?

JURY DUTY

The line moved fairly fast. The cause of the line? A security checkpoint and clearance. Just like at the airport. Now here's something I never expected. I can't believe there are people who go through that procedure every day before entering this building. Well, I felt safe, so that was good. I'm glad I opted not to wear a hat. I would've had to remove it, place it in the bin and walk through the security clearance all the while showing off my bad hair day. How embarrassing that would have been.

I made it. I'm actually sitting in the room where the rest of the jurors were waiting to be selected for different trials. I found a seat, pulled out my notebook and started writing. This is going to make a good chapter for my book, I thought. So much has already happened—and I haven't even entered a courtroom yet. They offered us free water and coffee while we sat and waited for our juror numbers to be called. I heard, "Number 255." That's me! I realized. Like a lottery, I've been selected. A sense of relief fell over me. I'm important. And most importantly—I made it to the right building, on the right day at the right time. Thank you, God.

While we waited, they gave us a questionnaire to complete. I thought they'd be yelling out questions at us over a microphone, narrowing down the selection process, like being selected for a beauty pageant. But wait! They were actual written questionnaires with 50 questions. It took me an hour to complete one. It felt like an SAT exam.

The questions, involving a medical malpractice suit, were interesting and the farther I went the more interesting they became. Oh, please let them choose me, I thought. I'm breaking out in a sweat here. Am I supposed to be sweating while completing this? There were more rules than I had to follow in a long time. Do something wrong? I dreaded the consequences.

The man at the podium ordered everyone to get into single file. Images of Catholic school entered my mind. The man continued, "We'll line you up by juror number. When everyone is called we'll walk single file to the elevators. Wait for me there. We are going to the third floor. When you exit, go to the end of the hall. The courtroom is on your left. Wait for me there."

What? Were we going to rush in and crash some kind of party? I didn't know, but wondered about his statement, "Wait for me there."

Okay, guy, I thought. I can do that. Sarcastically, I reflected on my thought, "If you can sit and you can wait, then you, too, are qualified to serve on jury duty." Okay, there's actually more involved than that, but I was beginning to feel like a dog in training with the same two commands repeated during my two weeks there: "Sit. Wait." I half-expected someone to say, "Good girl."

Finally, a voice said, "The trial will begin tomorrow morning at 9:30 AM."

Yes! Those words were music to my ears. I was being given the afternoon off. I wondered, does he know about my afternoon nap schedule? What a nice judge.

Driving home I smiled—and not just because of the early dismissal. I was glad I was following through with it. I'm doing my part as a U.S. citizen *and* reintegrating back into mainstream society, I thought. Nothing catastrophic happened on day one. I can do this!

The only courtroom experience I ever had was during my second hospitalization at the Mental Health Center.

Day two, and I was running on time—a good thing. I was in bed by 8:00 PM that Monday night. Was this how normal working people felt: drained, rushed and stressed every day? Geez, give me my pj's and bubble world any day over feeling like that.

JURY DUTY

The line to get into the District Courthouse went much faster on day two. I was even able to park a floor lower in the parking structure. Go, me! The courtroom in the District Courthouse was much larger and reminded me of one you'd see in a movie. It was very formal looking, yet the judge was laid back. I was surprised. I thought everything was going to be very proper and serious, and if you coughed everyone would stare and gasp, "How dare you?"

Fortunately, it wasn't that way, at all. I met several other people—interesting people who had no idea I had a mental illness—while we were in the waiting chambers. I felt more alive talking with normal people. It was one of the few times where I've been surrounded by them. I like it. I pretty much forget about my illness when I merely live each day. I'm just an ordinary person, too, who happens to have a mental condition for which I take medications so *I* can be normal.

And even though I wasn't selected to serve on a jury, I know in my heart that I would have made a good juror. Why? Because I'm honest, fair and a good listener. But I don't need a judge or lawyers to point that out to me—my friends tell me I have these good qualities. And who knows, down the road, I may be selected again to serve my country. I'd do it in a heartbeat because, as my therapist told me, I needed to take risks and grow, without letting my illness limit my life choices. She's so right.

ALWAYS

WHO?

Dr. Seuss. Yep. Dr. Seuss.
Such simple words that flow.
Has helped me grow…as a writer.
Writing books, I look back
How his writing kept me on track
Kept me wanting to read more
I couldn't wait to get to the bookstore

I started reading Dr. Seuss when I was a kid
He influenced me *so* much I couldn't get rid
Of the images and words on each page
…they were simply simple
…and I was hooked!

My favorite of his "Oh, the Places You'll Go"
I keep on my bookshelf
It's there to remind me
To lighten up on myself

Sometimes my days get busy, they do
Seems Dr. Seuss *always* knows what to do
"Open me up, open me up" he pleads
He always knows *exactly* what I need

With a chuckle and a smile
I turn each page
I'm so thankful this book was written for *any* age!

By Michelle Holtby ©2004

GET WELL, STAY WELL, MICHELLE

"When dealing with a problem: Think it through, and if there's something to do, do it right now. If there's nothing, forget it and don't worry, because no amount of worry will cure it."

—Carol Brennan

Decisions, decisions as I pray. My morning ritual prayer time brings me peace, calm and answers— answers to my "why's," "why not's" and "how's." I've had this private quiet time to myself for about a year. It's just something that I slowly integrated as one of my many self-care techniques. I awake every morning feeling anxious, with overwhelming feelings of tasks to do for the day and then, also, I replay the conversations of the past day or two that caused me distress. So this is the perfect time to set those things aside and just…breathe.

It's a technique I use in yoga every week—deep dish from the belly breathing, slowly and evenly and then exhaling at the same pace—but often I forget to do it on my own outside of class time. Somehow being in yoga class brings me calmness as soon as I walk in the door. I'm working on incorporating it into my daily life. I know it will give me more clarity with my decisions and help me to remain calm and not react to situations with lightning speed by verbally attacking the other person. Instead, I would like to see myself arriving at a place where I can listen to other people, process their information and then respond calmly—not like Animal from *The Muppets*.

Wow! That would be a welcome change from some of my current encounters. Strangers and acquaintances are safe—it's those closest to me, especially my parents, who are most susceptible to my bitter outbursts that seem to come from a hungry, untrained lioness. I don't draw blood, but my words have been known to resemble swords, being able to cut quick and deep, leaving the other person in shock. I'm not proud of this. My goal is to not drive away the people I love the most. Unfortunately, sometimes they're just around, and they happen to be the recipient of my behavior.

Retraining my brain to think before I speak is a relatively new concept for me. Be nice, Michelle. Play fair, I remind myself. I think of these and other positive, encouraging statements to help me stay on track.

I also rely on affirmation cards to help keep me focused on positive things. I have seven of them that I rotate through—one for each day of the week. Whenever my mind begins to wander to negative thoughts I recite the affirmation to myself until the thought passes. This has taken quite a huge amount of self-control and discipline, but the outcome has been completely worth it. My affirmation cards include the following statements:

"I let go. I let God." This affirmation is on my computer monitor in my office. Every time I glance downward it's like taking in a breath of peace.

"Success is a journey, not a destination." This one is

also in my office on a shelf. When I happen to look up in a certain direction it's in my line of vision. I can't help but look at it because I strategically placed it so I would see it whenever I reach for the dictionary or another reference book.

In addition to these cards, I have magnets, photos with inspiration quotes and a rock I keep on my desk in my room that simply says "Believe."

Having these things surrounding me is uplifting and I feel they also help keep me safe. Perhaps a little obsessive-compulsiveness plays into this, except I'm not placing any important attachment to them. I don't hold them or rub them for good luck. I just read them throughout the day. It's like I'm trying to reprogram my mind to block out negativity.

...

I'm broken. Looking at me from the outside you'd never see it. I'm a healthy, young woman who takes very good care of herself, on all levels. I don't drink or smoke, I usually get nine hours of sleep and I don't have promiscuous sex. I believe in God and have a close relationship with Him. I'm doing everything right. So, why is it that I can't give birth to a child?

One word—lithium. A simple, salt derivative that puts a grinding halt to even having the thought of a baby. And if I were to ignore my psychiatrist's advice and go forward with it, I'd be the "proud" mother of an extremely malformed fetus that would most likely die.

"Is it like Down's syndrome?" I asked my psychiatrist. I wanted to get *some* idea of what I was up against.

"It's incredibly worse, Michelle. And I don't advise you look it up on the internet. It's called *hydrops fetalis*. Just know that if you did choose to become pregnant, we'd definitely have to take you off lithium."

Lithium is my first and most reliable form of mood stabilizer to this day. Ironic that something that could work so well for me could kill someone else. Yes, sometimes life isn't fair. Perhaps this is why I've been petrified of becoming pregnant since I was 16. I wasn't diagnosed then, but the fear of becoming pregnant has been with me all these years. Attending a DBSA conference in 2002 and hearing speakers talk about pregnancy among women with mental illnesses confirmed my decision to not have a child. Having to change medications as soon as possible, close monitoring of me and the fetus and our stability level (my mental state and the fetus' physical state) would be too much to handle. There's too much at risk. And for what?

I'm reformed in my thinking. Until there is a cure for bipolar disorder no pregnancy for me. The end. The possibility of adoption is there, of course.

I'm beginning to see and hear that it's up to each couple whether they want children or not. It's not the family's requests and hopes. It's the couple's decision—a new concept for me.

I try not to feel jealous whenever I see friends with their children. I have to tell myself it's not some kind of competition where they're 'winners' and childless me is a 'loser.' Such thoughts are my negative mentality spiraling downward and taking over. It's ugly, draining and focuses on anyone who crosses my path. I lash out about the unfairness, blaming others, not being able to please everyone, not being perfect or like the rest of society.

What's wrong with me? Well, that's simple. I'm broken. Those thoughts kill me every time. My mental torture is my worst enemy.

I do wonder, why was I born with this illness? It's both

a curse and a gift. I can't have children. God, however, has given me the wonderful gift of writing and, who knows, perhaps one day I will write children's books. I remember what fun I had taking children's writing classes a couple of years ago. The creativity and fun allowed me to let my inner child out to play. It was very freeing. One of my favorites written for that class opens the third part of my memoir.

LIVING OUTSIDE
THE BUBBLE

"Sometimes you have to go backwards to go forward."
—Susan Zimmerman

Recently I read a well-known children's book at my Albuquerque Reads session called *The Hungry Little Caterpillar* by Eric Carle. It's a cute story that tells how a caterpillar turns into a butterfly.

This book actually applies to my life, as I'm now choosing to live it. For the longest time I was a shattered, scared and scarred young woman who was afraid to leave my home. Going out into the world seemed impossible. I thought I'd be trampled on by society because I didn't move or think as fast as everyone else. I was forced, more than chosen, to completely remove myself from the rat race of Corporate America—absolutely one of the best things I did for myself to maintain my sanity.

My cocoon was my parents' sunroom where I spent countless hours journaling and crying and just sitting. I resembled a statue, although if you were to touch me, I'm sure I would have crumbled into a million bipolar pieces. In *The Hungry Little Caterpillar,* the caterpillar knew when it was time to come out of his cocoon. He had grown as much as he could in that tiny little web home and when he emerged—well, I'm sure you know the rest—he was a beautiful butterfly that showed all the colors of the rainbow. And his wing span was huge. He wasn't afraid. It was his time to shine and go and explore and be free.

I resemble that butterfly. I, too, am no longer afraid to go out into the city and talk to people about my bipolar disorder. And I'm brave enough to be writing this book to share my experiences of living with a mental illness. I love to travel, whether it's a road trip or by plane. I want to travel around the country, maybe even the world, sharing my message of hope and my recovery from a mental illness. And I'm free to make my own daily choices how I want to live my life, how I choose to think and what I allow my brain to think about. With God as my guide, I trust Him every day to help keep me focused on my goals and to help keep my heart and ears open to His words.

Who knew that a children's book could resonate with my life? I believe we all have an inner child and that it's a good idea to regularly invite it to come out and play. The inner child keeps us young in spirit and thought. I know that I'm having a lot more fun when I incorporate joy into my day. There will *always* be work to do. For me, the fun stuff is what helps keep me balanced and is a reward for a job well done. So, grab a friend, a family member, or go alone. Try to do something nice for yourself each and every day.

I read somewhere recently that it takes 30 days to make or break a habit. I can testify to this. Writing my book every day takes time, dedication and perseverance. But I write at the same time each morning and have been doing it for several months. I didn't know it was going to become a habit. What began as writing for one hour has now increased to two hours. And the time just flies by.

I've come to realize that we may not know what talents we have and sometimes we find them in the most unlikely situations. But, it's up to us each day to choose how we're going to live our lives. Is it for ourselves? Or for God?

As much as possible, I choose to make my world a better place to live in. Not every day will be perfect, but there are things I can do to make other's lives easier or more enjoyable. I enjoy helping others. It gets myself out of "me" thinking and I completely focus on someone else's needs. I've noticed the more well I become, the more frequently I'm able to reach out and help others. I believe it helps to keep me in balance.

I certainly remember all the help I received when I couldn't take care of myself. I consider the present time in my life to be "paying it forward." And not because I have to, but because of the joy that's exchanged between me and another person when I do something nice. I believe that God has presented many opportunities for me to reach out and help others. I'm thankful for these opportunities and look forward to more coming my way.

TOOLS TO HEAL, HELP
AND CREATE

"Change is inevitable; growth is optional."
—Warren Spellell

I n addition to my self-care techniques, there are several other things that I have tried along my path to recovery. They are just ideas I share with you. They're listed in the order they came to my mind. I sat down one day with pen to paper and listed everything I could possibly think of that I've used as a tool to heal, help and create. Feel free to use or adapt them to meet your needs:

- Labyrinth (meditative walk)
- Private or group retreats at local Spirituality Center
- National Alliance on Mental Illness (NAMI) presentations
- DBSA guest speakers and activities
- One-hour daily naps
- Support network
- Slow down–live in the present moment
- Annual camping trips

- More space in your days—eliminating wearing a watch, for example, or not scheduling as much
- Make your priorities different from society (i.e. don't be so materialistic)
- Avoid crowds (do your shopping/errands during the mornings on Monday-Thursday)
- Take Yoga—I've done it nine years
- Take responsibility—for yourself and your illness
- Start new relationships–focus on positive people
- Take creative writing classes
- Have my morning coffee first—then talk (I'm not a morning person)
- Try traveling—especially road trips
- Hot tub soaks will relax you
- Monthly massages will relieve you of tensions
- Monthly Reiki sessions will put you in balance
- Try Wellness Recovery Action Plan (WRAP) Plan for maintaining your recovery success
- Consider your purpose of life clearly defined over time
- Try the arts (I became a certified graphic de-signer/freelance writer)
- Avoid waste or excess: "Use what you have"
- Cherish your friendships more (quality vs. quantity)
- A Mental Health Center treatment team—a psychia-trist, nurse and therapist—was successful for me
- Keep snacks in purse and in car to prevent low blood sugar
- Take water wherever you go to alleviate cotton mouth (dry mouth)
- Try volunteering. I participate in Albuquerque Reads (program that teaches kindergarteners how to read)

TOOLS TO HEAL

- Avoid malls, which are overwhelming, especially on weekends. I prefer outside shops to reduce claustrophobia. I leave the mega-stores for my parents.
- Keep things small and simple. Too many choices stresses me out!
- Have time in nature with God.
- Read self-help books
- Read faith-based novels
- Do church "shopping" for the right match for your needs
- Get some fresh air–take a walk at a park or in your neighborhood
- Have some daily alone time to reflect and relax
- Make time with others–coffee, take a walk, or do a hobby together

I began this list several years ago. As time goes by, I'm sure I'll add more to it. The list includes things that have helped me. Perhaps they will be a starting place for ideas of your own. One good outcome about having bipolar disorder is that people who have it are very creative. I don't know of any other illnesses that have such positive attributes. Have fun with the list above. But most importantly, make it your own. Perhaps start with one or two ideas and then let it grow from there.

The items I listed were not given to me by anyone. They just came to me over time. They will not guarantee that you will be cured, but they will enhance your recovery process. It'll give you the opportunity to step outside your illness and little by little rejoin "regular" people. Please remember to have fun no matter how you decide to use this list.

COPING TECHNIQUES

"Truly, it is in the darkness that one finds the light, so when we are in sorrow, then this light is nearest of all to us."
—Meister Eckhart

I've never liked the word "coping." It makes me think of drowning or barely hanging on. The word didn't even enter my vocabulary until I was diagnosed. I choose to call my coping techniques "self-care techniques." It sounds more positive and upbeat, like me.

While some of these techniques I picked up from others, like at DBSA meetings, most of them I came up with on my own. I think how each of us chooses to live with our illness is unique. And to have a successful recovery, we need to find those things that best match our needs and incorporate them into our lives.

One of the first things I learned about living with my illness was that I needed an outlet to express how I felt about things—anything that was on my mind and eating away at me. I began to journal—nothing fancy, just a regular spiral bound notebook I found in my desk and a pen. Whatever I wanted to say, I wanted it to be permanent. No erasing, no going back, which meant no using pencils. Just like this illness. Permanent. My options were to stay stuck or move forward. And believe me, I may as well have been moving a bull elephant across Africa with the amount of physical, mental and emotional energy it took at the beginning of my journaling days.

I would sit in the sunroom, turn the notebook to a blank page, put the pen to paper and in-stream-of-consciousness, write anything and everything that wanted to show its ugly head on paper. I wasn't afraid or ashamed. Journaling was incredibly therapeutic. Because I didn't feel I had adequate time to confide in my psychiatrist–and my parents lacked the knowledge about my illness so couldn't really help me out–it was up to me and my journal to get my recovery process started. What I wrote often didn't make any sense. My grammar and sentence structure would have sent my English teacher into cardiac arrest. It didn't matter. I wasn't planning on showing this notebook to anyone. It has been my emotional dumping station for six-and-a-half years, and it's been incredibly helpful.

It was a plain notebook. I felt that pretty words were meant to be written in fancy, decorative journals. It was a down-and-dirty word writing time, though, and plainness was absolutely appropriate. I didn't want anything coming between me and my thoughts. If I wrote a bunch of ugly cuss words in a journal with, "Reach for Your Dreams" written on the cover, it just didn't seem appropriate. Dreams? What dreams? I was living a nightmare!

I didn't know where my writing would lead me. I just knew that every day I needed to do it. I began about six months after I was discharged and had experienced months of depression. Writing actually made me feel a little bit better. Writing has helped me sort through my feelings—mainly anger, loss and frustration and the direction my life was heading in—what felt like the land of eternal unknowingness, especially during the first several years. I never reread what I wrote until I began writing my book.

I'm at a point now in my recovery process where I feel emotionally strong enough to face the words on the notebook pages written by a broken girl not so long ago.

If writing isn't your thing, perhaps an audio tape recording would be beneficial. I must admit, talking is faster, but for me it was a matter of getting pen to paper and "burning some rubber."

My talk time came in the form of a support group. About a year passed by before I decided to join the Depression and Bipolar Support Alliance (DBSA). There were many people who walked into my life during the four years I was a member. I made some good friends, and I felt it was the one place where I could open up and speak freely about what was on my mind. What surprised me was that most of the things I had shared, many of those people had experienced.

I received incredible help, comfort and acceptance from them. We were all in this together. It was the first time I felt I truly belonged. With their kind, supportive words, they handled my heart with care. I miss those friends, but I am thankful for the time they were in my life. I believe that people are in our lives for a reason, a season or a lifetime and, in this case, it was for a very special reason. They helped me heal and learn how to accept my illness through their words and actions and the way they lived their lives. They taught me about self-acceptance and forgiveness—for myself and others.

DBSA became much more than a weekly support group for me. They had monthly guest speakers on a variety of interesting, relevant topics. They went on social outings, which I liked, because it got me out of the support-group frame of mind, and I got to know people as people. We went to concerts, bowling, movies, restaurants, hikes and various other places. I miss those things.

One thing that I stopped doing was wearing a watch. Time no longer mattered to me. I had nowhere to go, no schedule to adhere to, so what was the point? If I needed to know the time, there was usually a clock nearby, either in my car or wherever I was going. It was freeing in a way. Working in advertising, time was of the essence. Checking the time almost felt like an obsessive-compulsive requirement. I felt like I'd been ultimately freed from the Corporate World by making an outward statement that I, Michelle Holtby, chose to no longer let my life be dictated by time. It was anxiety-provoking at first and it took a couple years for my watch tan line to disappear, but ultimately it became freeing. I was no longer operating on "this world time" but on God's time. It felt like a vacation from the 8-5 Corporate World and from people's expectations of where and when I needed to be at certain times.

I've only recently begun wearing watches again, but they're mainly to accessorize. They resemble bracelets more than a timepiece. And I like it this way. The only time I make sure to wear a watch is when I travel. Being late for a plane or seminar would not be good.

Reading the daily newspaper and watching the evening news were both choices that I have eliminated from my life after my diagnosis. Although I believe it's my fragile brain that prevents me from being able to cope with bad news, I'm sure there's plenty of other people without a mental illness who'd rather not read about mayhem and disaster day-in and day-out. It's taxing on one's mental state. And if the first thing we choose to read over breakfast is bad news, then what does that say for the rest of our day? I believe that people have enough personal problems and sharing some optimism would do everyone a bit of good.

Okay, I'm stepping off my soapbox now.

I received my credit card sized affirmation cards as a gift from my yoga instructor. I saw a couple of them on her computer at the yoga studio and she printed me my very own set. I put one on my bedroom mirror, another on my bathroom mirror, computer monitor, on my desk, in my wallet and the dash of my car. I consider them to be little "pick me ups." They say "I live in the moment," "I love and approve of myself," "I am free to be," "I am at peace with my own feelings," "I am perfect, whole and complete," and "I am always Divinely protected and guided." I've had them for more than a year and they're great little reminders that God is watching over me.

I would say the biggest surprise out of my whole bipolar disorder experience is the wonderful gifts I have received. "Gifts, from an illness?" you may be asking yourself. "How is this humanly possible?"

When I was first diagnosed I said it was the absolute worst thing that ever happened to me. Now I say that having bipolar disorder is the absolute best thing that's ever happened to me. I feel like I have been given a second chance from God to do things His way. As it turns out, doing things His way is surprisingly easier.

I feel more connected to Him in the past couple of years. I'm led by Him each day when I begin my mornings by praying. I talk to Him throughout the day. He guides me. I turn to Him for advice on dating, on getting along with my parents, and I completely trust that He will bring people and opportunities into my life when appropriate.

I feel I have self-respect. I'm learning that while not everyone may like me it's not up to me to change their minds and convince them that I'm a worthy person of knowing. Life's too short. I choose to surround myself with positive, optimistic people who aren't afraid to live.

I think that losing everything I had—health, home and people—taught me how much I have to be thankful for. I feel things much more deeply. I definitely have become a more sensitive person. I may be the first to cry in an argument or lash out in bitter anger at a loved one. I don't know where the intensity of these emotions comes from, but they're real and they're mine and I wouldn't have it any other way.

EDUCATION

"Healing is embracing what is most feared; healing is opening what has been closed, softening what has hardened into obstruction, healing is learning to trust life."
                                             —Jeanne Achterberg

A n important part of my continuing healing process is education for myself and others. Since I've been diagnosed, I continue to learn new things about my illness. I've attended DBSA and NAMI national conventions. Attending these conferences has given me hope, an opportunity to connect with others who are on their own healing path and information that I can share with others when I return home.

I think the main reason I'm so interested in educating myself is because it encourages me that discovering a cure becomes much closer to reality with each passing year. I have the utmost faith that a cure for bipolar disorder will be discovered during my lifetime. And I look forward to the day when I won't need to take medications to balance my mood.

It seems like such an obscure thought right now. Would I act the same, meaning the way I am now, but without medications or would I experience other mood swings? I don't dwell on these thoughts too often. Right now I'm fully engrossed in the education process and helping as many people as possible who suffer from this very common and potentially debilitating illness.

I'm also a big book reader. I believe that knowledge is power. I've read many books about bipolar disorder, especially during the first couple of years after I was diagnosed. Many of the answers that others couldn't provide, I found in self-help books. At the back of this book I've listed some of the books I recommend as insightful reading.

I want to empower others by sharing what I've learned. Over the years, I've learned that the more I know about my illness, the more I heal. I choose not to let my illness run my life. New books about bipolar disorder are always being published, and I make a habit of checking the local bookstores and library regularly to find them.

Often, I will check out a new book at the library and, if I really like it, I'll buy a copy at the bookstore. I have several friends who have bipolar disorder. If I think it'll help them, I'll tell them about the book because I want others to better understand this brain disorder. It's made our friendships stronger and we're better able to understand each other.

I'd also like to say that I don't primarily focus on self-help or memoir books about bipolar disorder. Yes, they are very important, but I prefer to be a well-rounded reader, so I read books about different topics. I mentioned earlier in my book, *The Artist's Way* by Julia Cameron, a book about tapping into creativity. I didn't know what was going to come out of reading this book, but I kept an open mind.

During the 12 weeks it took me to read it, I felt like I was exploring a new part of me—my spiritual side. I drank up what I read, completing all the written exercises, going on my artist dates and coming out a better person. No church or person or vacation could have possibly made the positive changes that occurred inside me. It has been one of my favorite books and remains in my permanent book collection.

My hope is that by writing this book, others will be inspired to share their story. People have told me how brave I am, letting skeletons out of the closet, but honestly, it feels like the right time to do that. And I feel I have such purpose in sharing my story. A few people were ahead of me in writing their memoirs, but there's one main difference—hope. I'm telling my story with a purpose. Nothing could be more exposed or raw or healing as telling you my story from my heart. The way I talk is the way I write, so you can think of this book as having one long conversation with me.

To start a new trend of hopeful memoirs would be absolutely fantastic. It's one thing to share your personal story with a few close friends, but to completely trust and open your heart to share your story with the world—well, I'd say that takes some guts. But for me, what I've received in return has been surprisingly wonderful. I'm not here to preach about it, but just to say "think about it." It could possibly be one of the best things you can do for yourself in your healing process.

As I mentioned in an earlier chapter, I've been giving "In Our Own Voice" (IOOV) presentations for four years now. Sharing my story with the inpatients is very humbling for me. It's such a fine line to walk between being mentally well or sick. Giving my bi-monthly presentations is a reality check-in for me and a reminder to keep taking good care of myself. Yes, even with my treatment team— my psychiatrist, therapist, parents, and friends—I still place 99 percent of the responsibility to take care of myself on me.

To stay well is something I choose every day. I focus

on activities and being around people who support me, encourage me and look out for my overall well-being. I'm extremely paranoiac of being hospitalized again. My manic episodes, while they are partially humorous, are for the most part quite frightening. To not be able to tell reality from fantasy is frightening, very confusing and downright nerve-wracking. But to have no inhibitions or cares in the world and feel like a young child was fun. I was really lucky that nothing bad happened to me. God was definitely watching over me. I am a *very* lucky young lady. I was properly diagnosed, hospitalized and treated by the caring staff at the UNM Mental Health Center. Many mentally ill are taken directly to jail.

And this is why I share my story—so that others won't have to go through what I did. But even if you've been diagnosed for a long time, perhaps my words will wake up something inside you, to move you forward with your life, to make one, small positive change, psychologists tell us takes only 30 days of continuous practice to see that change turn into a habit.

One of my goals upon completing this book is to travel around the country. I would really enjoy sharing my story with others, connecting with them and hearing their stories. I think that's the reason why we're all here—to help each other and make life's journey easier and more enjoyable. I know that I've gone through enough emotional pain for a lifetime. I've come through to the other side now, and I feel I have so much to be grateful for. I want to share this with others.

Don't get me wrong, though, my life is definitely not perfect. As a matter of fact, I've had to completely redesign my life to accommodate my illness. But, I wouldn't have it any other way. I don't miss being in the Corporate World and working grueling hours, overtime, being caught in traffic, and having a humongous mortgage payment.

Nothing is wrong with any of those things. I just choose not to expose myself to that lifestyle any longer. It's very stressful for me. I had to reeducate myself and reprioritize things in my life. There's no manual (unless you count this book) on how to live with bipolar disorder. No manual such as *Welcome to the World of Bipolar Disorder* was given to me by my psychiatrist after I was diagnosed. I wish. Just like parents with a newborn could probably use a manual, I could have, too. No, I had to teach myself and learn on my own about what works, what doesn't and what never will. Living and learning about this bipolar thing is damn hard and sometimes it just sucks beyond anything I've ever known.

One thing that has piqued my curiosity for the past several months is each person's level of wellness. I believe there are different degrees to which each person with bipolar disorder is capable of functioning. I consider myself to be a highly functioning person with this illness. I have several friends who are also highly functioning. It got me to thinking that why aren't there more people who are able to obtain this level of functioning as well? What qualities determine whether a person will survive or thrive with this illness?

Well, I don't have a background in biology, chemistry, neurology, psychology or even sociology. But I do have an extensive amount of bipolar disorder experience. So, here's the formula that I came up with for a successful recovery with bipolar disorder:

Male/Female (equal)

- Environment
- Medications-compliant/effective

- Treatment team interaction/support
- Stress level
- Family
- Education level
- Age of bipolar onset
- Spirituality
- Optimist vs. Pessimist
- Involvement in Recovery
- Therapy-group/individual
- Time outdoors
- Daily Routine

VALUES

"We make a living by what we get. But we make a life by what we give."

—Cheryl Kilbourn

Simplicity is key. My, how my values have changed and evolved over the past several years. Trading in my Corporate America way of living for the simple life is probably one of the best things I've chosen to do.

Money is important, but having time to do and be whatever I want holds much more weight for me. Time is such a precious commodity, and I'm so thankful that most of my day is filled with activities I want to do, and not what I *have* to do. My time reflects my values. Everything I do flows from ideas I have. And sometimes these ideas come from God.

Attending Albuquerque Reads once a week is an example. So is my morning prayer time and having a quiet breakfast with Tigger in the sunroom. I try not to take anything for granted. I know how hard I had to work at creating this life that I love and how quickly it could change. I'm thankful I don't have to get ready each morning and rush out the door. I can watch the robins and doves in the backyard as they perch on or splash around in our birdbath.

227

BIPOLAR NO MORE

Looking out the sunroom windows is like looking at a picture. It's very soothing, and I look forward to it each morning. Everything is quiet. I value starting every day this way. I have nothing to race off to because I've made it a priority to pace myself and not schedule activities until the afternoon. I've grown to enjoy hanging out in my pj's writing this book. Comfort, quiet and Tigger by my side. This is heaven for me.

I also try to limit how much TV I watch. I prefer to read. Whether it's a good faith-based novel or Oprah magazine, I try to envelop my world with positive, uplifting things. The movies I watch are usually comedies and, yes, I even watch kids' animated films such as "Alvin and the Chipmunks." Even within children's movies, there's an element of adulthood. And, of course, when "Horton Hears a Who" comes to the dollar theater I plan on seeing it simply because I'm a Dr. Seuss fan.

Speaking of the dollar movie theater—there are many things in my life I've had to adapt to, including how I choose to spend money. Again, this revolves around my values. With our beautiful weather here most of the year, there's nothing like stopping at a yard sale to chat with the neighbors and pick up a treasure or two.

I rarely visit the local shopping center. The parking situation and high prices keep me away. When I think I need something, I look through my closet first and assess if there's something that will work. If not, then I'll visit the local thrift store or consignment store. I'm so thankful there are several of these stores in town.

When I was working in Corporate America I didn't even notice these stores when I drove past them. Now, I scout them out. It's amazing what people donate. Some things I've purchased still have the original sales tags on them! It's the little things in life that make me happy. And the things I purchase I know are one of a kind. I like being unique. I do admit that I go to the shopping malls when there are clearance sales—especially on shoes. Fifty to 75 percent off—I enjoy seeing how much money I can save on things—it's like Christmas.

And when I need help, I'm not afraid to ask. Whether it's seeing my therapist once a week or talking with my good friend Lori in California. I just stay tuned into what I need. Talk therapy helps sometimes, but sometimes I just need to get out of the house and take a nice, long walk through the neighborhood to clear my mind.

It feels like there's a boot in my head that's kicking and stomping on negative thoughts as they arise. Sometimes I actually get a headache. Life's too short to dwell on negative things. If something isn't working for me then I definitely take action. I'm very much a proactive person.

It's upsetting when my world isn't in balance because it's all I think about until things get remedied. There are days, even weeks, that can go by where I'm in balance. I remember these times and strive to return to them. I'm definitely a "fixer" and I rarely give up—which is not always a good thing. Knowing when to quit and when to move on is a constant stressor for me. Being a quitter was never taught to me as a young child.

I squeeze the life out of a problem, twisting and turning it and banging it on the ground and stomping on it and yelling and crying at it to make it better. My conflict resolution skills, I admit, are not the cream of the crop. If none of these methods work, then I go pick up a copy of a Dr. Phil's relationship book and look for answers.

Books may not have worked with Josh, but they seem to help *me*. Maybe for Josh, it was the right author, but the wrong time and perhaps the wrong person. I'm big on reading books for advice or suggestions. I think there's a wealth of knowledge out there and if I can read about something that someone else has gone through to help ease my pain, then all the better. I believe we're all here to help each other, and there are different ways this is made possible.

While saving money is a high priority for me, there are some things that I will not skimp on: proper care for Tigger—vet visits, groomer, dog food and bones. Only the best for my little dog child. I think I treat him better than some people treat their own kids. To me, he is more human than doglike. He helps keep me in balance with daily walks, listening to my problems, licking my tears away and keeping me company when no one else is around. He's my little four-legged guardian angel. Just like I don't skimp on my healthcare, his healthcare is the same. We help take care of each other.

I'm very thankful for the people in my life and try to show them in various ways how much I appreciate and value them. My parents' unending support, doing activities with others and talking with my friends are all an integral part of my staying well.

Although my friends I had prior to my diagnosis are no longer in my life—their choice—the ones who are now in my life are priceless. They've taught me so much about myself, including acceptance, love, understanding and not to take myself so seriously. They want to be around me for who I am, not what I have to offer (it used to be about material things and in some cases, sex.) I'm not embarrassed to say that. I was a completely different person before my diagnosis. And, unfortunately, I had to go through a lot of ugliness and personal growth to get to where I'm at today.

Today I feel incredibly blessed. I feel God's presence continuously throughout the day. I know what I need to do to take care of myself. Some days are low-energy days and I just need to give myself a break, allow myself to slow down and not stress about taking on too many activities. I know eventually I'll bounce back in a couple of days and be highly productive again. I'm very fortunate being self-employed, so I can take personal days and am able to pace myself. It's a give and take, kind of like being a rubber band.

I can be stretched only so far before I have to retract, or in my case, regroup. If not, I snap and believe me, that is not pretty. It comes out as sarcasm, crying, isolation and having really low energy. Even after seven years I still experience bipolar highs and lows, but with medication they're more tolerable and they don't last as long as a full-blown episode would. Thank goodness for that.

What else do I value? I value my ability to write. I honestly never knew I was a writer until about a year ago when I began putting this book together. It began merely as daily journaling to dump out my feelings. I didn't even write complete sentences. Just thoughts. But with time, I pieced things together, created topics and thought, "You know, I think I have enough material here to write a book. There is some good stuff here I think people could benefit from reading."

So, day by day, I chipped away and organized my extensive stack of notebooks into topics and then gradually began filling in the gaps. It didn't even seem like work. It seems like the most absolute right thing I've ever done with my life. The words flow onto the computer screen like chocolate silk, smoothly and sweetly helping to heal the deep wounds in my soul. I know that God is behind this project. I have bipolar disorder and God is working through me, so I can share my story with others and help ease or eliminate their pain. Yes, of course, I wish I didn't have to go through what I did, but I did it—and I'm not only surviving, I'm thriving. I'm only able to live this way with His help.

After all I've been through, I value each breath, each beautiful sunset, moments with Tigger and holding someone's hand, to name a few things. They may be just the little moments, but these little moments are what make up a lifetime. I pray that experiencing this illness is the worst thing that I'll ever have to endure. It was a surprise to discover how much stronger a person it made me. And there's nothing like going through a tragedy to reprioritize your values. Suddenly breathing in the smell of spring or dancing just because you can means a whole lot more. I only wish that it didn't take having to go through such a tragic event for me to appreciate life's little things. But, I suppose it was my huge wakeup call from God. And believe me, it was much stronger than any cup of coffee I've *ever* drunk!

GIVING BACK

"Money will come when you are doing the right thing."
—Mike Phillips

I think somewhere deep down inside me I knew that I was a giver. I still am, actually. I've volunteered for a variety of things through the years—some were long-term projects while others lasted for just an afternoon or a weekend. Somehow, I forgot that good feeling that goes with being a giver. It's different from being in love or cuddling with a puppy. For me, it's an inner, glowing feeling that energizes me down to my toes. I feel that all is well in my world. I wish I could carry this feeling with me all the time. And I think I've figured out how.

There's giving of money and there's giving of time. Which is more important? I'm not convinced that one is better than the other. I remember before I was diagnosed and I was working in advertising, I earned a really nice paycheck. But my connection to money was odd. I hoarded it. I wished for more. I wished for more *things* in my life because I thought these things would bring me happiness. Oh, how twisted my thoughts were on this subject. I went to church off and on, and I gave adequate donations but something was different. I didn't feel good about giving money at church, and I didn't feel bad for not giving enough. I felt—nothing. Empty.

Is this how it works? People donate money to their chosen church every week regardless of how they feel about it?

I didn't wonder if I was helping to pay someone's salary, pay for copying the bulletin for the following week or even paying some part of upkeep of the church building. I just knew that it was my duty to give money to the church. My parents did it the entire time I was growing up. Now it was my turn to participate. But it didn't feel good at all. It was rather disappointing. No warm fuzzies.

I thought, maybe if I give more money then I'll get a positive response. I gave more and felt absolutely the same. It was downright frustrating. It wasn't until after I lost my health, job, boyfriend, home and dignity did I find out that there are other ways to give. It was very humbling, yet refreshing, to know there was an alternative.

I've been rather limited on funds, so giving my time wins. I think it's something that's within each of us. I remember several years ago volunteering to help build homes for Habitat for Humanity. What an amazing experience. Without so much as a hammer-in-hand experience, I was given a crash course in putting up sheetrock. I didn't even know what sheetrock was. But there I was, jumping in with willingness to help. And at the end of the day, to see what a group of people could accomplish—building a home for a family that otherwise didn't have a safe, adequately sized place to live in—was amazing. I went home exhausted, and I had a few blisters, but that didn't stop the good feeling of helping someone in need. In my heart, I knew I'd do it again if the opportunity arose.

For the past four years I've had the wonderful opportunity to be a part of NAMI's "In Our Own Voice" program.

GIVING BACK

The people I met have been amazing. And being able to share my story has allowed me the opportunity to continue to heal. Never before have I participated in something that was a win-win situation. Before I give a presentation I say a silent prayer in my car and ask God that He allow me to reach at least one person in the audience. And this usually happens. I feel His grace as He gives me the right words to connect with the audience and give them hope that they, too, can have a successful recovery. I am living proof that coming out of the other side of bipolar disorder can be a positive experience. I am thankful that God has helped me get over my terror of public speaking so I *can* reach people.

Recently, I had the opportunity to attend a weekend of Clarus at our church. I must admit, I'm not the most savvy person when it comes to understanding the Bible, but that didn't matter. What caught and kept my attention was the pastor's enthusiasm of what he was speaking about. His voice boomed at times and was barely an audible whisper at others. He made his points with carefully chosen words. He was passionate about what he was doing. He was doing exactly what God had intended him to do here on earth.

I thought to myself "Wow, this man's passionate."

I don't remember the last time I heard a speaker like him. I took notes. But the fluctuation in his voice tone and the words he chose were like special songs that were written for us to hear. It was as if each topic was a new song for us to experience. To open up our ears and hearts and really hear the music—the message—he was sharing. It was like watching a conductor of a symphony. His arms punched the air with the points he made, and he removed and replaced his eye glasses numerous times, putting them on to emphasize points from the Bible and removing them to talk to the audience.

I think I speak with passion. Maybe toned down a little,

but I believe the truth and rawness of my personal story reaches people. I feel God working through me when I give my presentations. It feels so right. I feel energized knowing that I can help someone. Maybe I can make some part of their journey a little easier to bear or perhaps I can give someone an opportunity to view something in a different way. I enjoy helping people. I never knew it would be of this magnitude, but as long as God continues to guide me along this particular path, I will keep doing His work.

Some people may wonder, "How in the world do you still believe in God, much less want to help Him?" The answer to that is *time*. Believe me, when I was first diagnosed with my horrific illness, I wanted nothing to do with God. My life was going along just fine, I was successful and happy (so I thought).

Then God comes along and rips my life in half and slaps me in the face with bipolar disorder illness. The last person I wanted in my life was Him. I was mad and lost and frustrated and lonely, and I didn't know why. I'm not a bad person. I didn't ask for this. Time brings healing, though. For me, it took several years and it was a very slow process. I had to learn to trust Him again. I cried about this a lot, and I wrote in my journal, "How and why should I trust someone who wrecked my world?"

Slowly, my heart started to heal. For several years after I was diagnosed I couldn't give anything. The light to my heart was turned off. Inside me, it was cold and black. I couldn't even take care of myself. I relied heavily on my parents to provide everything on a physical level I needed, to make it through each day. Chewing my food and getting dressed felt like mountains to climb. Everything required so much energy and time. I felt like a run-down flash light that was in desperate need of being recharged. "This little light of mine" was not shining too brightly those days.

Even crying and blowing my nose took so much effort. I didn't care if the snot ran down over my mouth and dribbled onto my shirt. No one was around to watch me. I was a mess and I didn't care.

When did I stop caring? I think I had to hit complete bottom to begin my ascent to healing. Fortunately, God doesn't judge us, even during our darkest times. And for me, the six months following my diagnosis were my darkest times. I think I had to experience that dark time of my life to start my journey to healing. Gradually, over the period of several years, I began to gain strength and energy, and I had a joy for life again. It wasn't one thing or one person that did it, but rather, a collective group of things.

I slowly began to reach a level of balance in my life. The inner thawing of my heart took time. And with time, came forgiveness and understanding. It's definitely not a process to be rushed and it's different for each person. But, for me, before giving could occur, whether it's time, talents or money, I had to forgive myself and stop blaming myself for my illness. The conclusion I came to is that it was not my fault and it lifted a huge weight off my heart.

Giving presentations at the UNM Mental Health Center has been something I've been doing since January 2007. It's been important for me for a long time to find a way to give back to this hospital. My psychiatrist, nurse and therapist have helped me so much. I consider it paying it forward. I do it because I want to, not because I have to. I look forward to giving IOOV presentations twice a month. I want to make available to others what wasn't available for me when I was initially hospitalized there seven years ago. It wasn't anyone's fault. The program just didn't yet exist in Albuquerque.

I think the running theme through my life is that I experience or learn things and then I receive the meaning of it and it makes some sense. Sometimes I wish we could request manuals, like Cliff Notes from God, about things we're experiencing. Then maybe some of our pain could be eliminated. I guess it would be called prayer. Whoa! I just answered my own dilemma!

I've mentioned another organization that I wholeheartedly believe in: Albuquerque Reads. I've been a volunteer for two years, helping to teach kindergarteners how to read. They enter the program with none or very minimal reading capability. But Albuquerque Reads is a wonderful program that's highly structured, and it's proven that by the end of the school year, the little 5-year-olds will be reading to us tutors.

I believe that teaching a child to read is priceless. I am so fortunate that I have the weekly time available and personal enjoyment of reading to share with two children each Monday. I'm thankful to be a part of helping to reduce illiteracy in our city. I look forward to returning next fall.

I love seeing their faces light up when they're able to sound out a word and gradually build up their reading skills to read an entire book to me. It's amazing.

I know my limits. I know what I can handle. And right now I'm able to help two kids each week learn how to read. I'm thankful God has given me the time and patience to help these children. I have played a very important part in helping these children learn a skill they'll use for the rest of their lives.

I'm fully engrossed when I'm teaching. Whatever else may be on my plate doesn't matter. It's swept aside and I'm completely present for these kids. I'm certain that many of them don't get adequate attention from their family and reading isn't at the top of the list of their family activities.

But for me, it was my dad's love of reading that got passed down to me. Every night after dinner, I read out loud to my dad while he washed the dishes. I remember it so vividly. I can even smell the clean scent of dishwater bubbles and hear my dad's voice when I spelled out a word I didn't know to him. He didn't even have to turn around. I'd spell out the word. He'd pause for a moment and tell me what it was. Then I'd go back and reread the entire sentence with the new word added to my vocabulary bag. I loved reading. Beginning when I was 5, I did this for several more years. It's interesting which memories stick with us.

I still enjoy reading. My hope is that by helping the kindergarteners learn to read, they'll remember the weekly tutoring sessions and develop an enjoyment of reading. Albuquerque Reads didn't exist when I was in elementary school. It's a relatively new program in our city and it's available only at a handful of public schools.

Fortunately, I don't think about my bipolar disorder when I'm helping the kids. They certainly don't know I have bipolar disorder. As a matter of fact, no one knows. I look and I act just like everyone else. There's no need for me to broadcast my illness.

Ironically, though, if I was never diagnosed I probably wouldn't have become involved in the reading program. Why? I'm more humble and more willing to give of my time, talents and energy now. Before I was diagnosed, it was all about me—The Michelle Show. It's amazing what a diagnosis can do to your outlook on life. I don't recommend rushing out and getting a diagnosis, but if you have one, especially a mental one, I think you know exactly what I mean.

I had to go backwards to move forward with my life. In other words, I had to lose everything in order to get some perspective on my life. And, did God give me a huge dose of perspective! But whenever I'm driving out of the school parking lot after a tutoring session, I feel good about myself. I helped a child learn something new. And that's something you can't put a dollar amount on.

...

My latest endeavor is the SMART™ program. I created it after realizing the limitations to the "In Our Own Voice" program. It consists of five things: Support, Medication, Awareness, Reaching Out and Treatment (SMART™). It's a presentation that embraces these five key elements to a continuing successful recovery.

I believe much good will come from this program. I would very much embrace the opportunity to travel around the country, even the world, sharing this program with people. It's not just intended for the mentally ill, but for everyone. My goal is to promote hope and recovery and education. Every day I choose to "walk the walk." It keeps me well and focused on maintaining my wellness. I make it a daily priority to take care of myself mentally, emotionally, physically and spiritually. If there are problems cluttering my mind I handle them in four ways: I pray it out, walk it out, talk it out or write it out.

I think of SMART™ like a tree growing with several branches. But before any branches are encouraged to grow, there must be a deep root to keep it steady, focused and strong. I believe the root is my connection with God. When the branches sway, I want to know that my root, or my core, will be there for me through everything. Of course, proper watering is also essential for the overall health of the tree— which implies spending time with God daily in some spiritual way. For me, it's my morning prayer time. I read a passage from my prayer book, do some yoga stretches, prepare my mind for the day's activities and ask God to be with me throughout the day.

Support is the first branch of the program. It includes family, friends, pets, DBSA, NAMI, psychiatrists, psychotherapy and books. What we choose to include in our support system is as unique as each of us. I have had all of these elements in my support portion throughout my recovery. As length and thickness of tree branches vary, so too have these various elements remained in my life and impacted my recovery. Some are still an integral part of my recovery, such as my psychiatrist and NAMI. Others have changed as my wellness level shifts, such as the friends who have come in and out of my life over the years. I choose to have a few really close friends who have been a part of my main support system, as well as my parents and Tigger. I believe that with the right support system a long-term strong, successful recovery is definitely possible.

Medication is the second key ingredient to a successful recovery. While I don't discuss the medications I'm currently taking, I do know that they have been an integral part in helping to balance my moods and keep me well. And just like we each have different eye and hair color, our medications are prescribed for our very specific symptoms. Oh, how nice it would be if bipolar disorder treatment were more of a cookie cutter approach, meaning find some combination that works for everyone with this illness. And minimal side effects would be nice, too.

But that's not quite the case yet. Frustrating at the beginning, I thought my psychiatric medications would work just like taking an aspirin. Wait a few minutes and then your headache is gone. Not so with psychiatric meds. No one told me it could take months for my meds to kick in. I'm patient, but come on! After my second hospitalization, six months of being mentally miserable was no Disneyland for me. I began to think that nothing was going to work–

talk about anxiety provoking. But, just as I took multivitamins for my body every day, my parents watched to make sure I also took my psychiatric meds. And I did. I was paranoiac something bad would happen if I stopped.

I remember looking at my little entourage of pills all lined up by size and color and talking to each one before swallowing it: "Please work, little pink pill. Help my brain feel better. You know where to swim to once you're inside me." Down the hatch.

It took a couple of years before I became completely comfortable taking my meds. My side-effects are minimal, thank goodness: dry mouth and constipation. The side-effects fluctuates throughout the year, but I find that if I drink enough water, exercise daily and eat fruits and vegetables, my body remains happy.

Awareness is the third key ingredient. The Wellness Recovery Action Plan (WRAP) has been an integral part of my recovery process. It's a document that I, my parents, psychiatrist, nurse, Pete and Lisa all have. It looks like a term paper (I'm very thorough) and is like a health insurance policy. It includes specific things to make sure I stay well, what happens when things start to fall apart, what to do in a crisis situation, and the steps to take after a hospitalization to get me back on track.

WRAP was developed by Mary Ellen Copeland. You can access this online at: www.mentalhealthrecovery.com and you can create your own plan. I made my plan to give me peace of mind knowing that if I think I'm starting to slip, what can be done to stop it and get me back on track. I created the plan a couple years after my second hospitalization, and it has been an immensely helpful tool to keep me well. Over the years, I've updated it as new triggers or ways of coping enter my life. It's the best way I know for my loved ones to understand my illness and how they can best help me when I'm not feeling well.

Reaching Out is the fourth ingredient. I believe that once you are at a certain point in your recovery process it's a natural tendency to want to give back. That's what happened to me and why I volunteer to do IOOV presentations. It took a few years for me to get to this step, and I know it's an ongoing integral part of my recovery. I never realized that sharing my personal story of living with a mental illness was going to be a healing experience for me. But it is, and it continues to be an important part of my overall well being.

Treatment is the final element, or branch, in the SMART™ program. While psychiatrists are important, there are other forms of treatment that I've been fortunate to receive during my recovery. I've participated in psychotherapy a couple of times in my recovery process. Talk therapy has been a very helpful addition to my meds and my psychiatrist. Having someone who understands me and who doesn't judge me has been really important.

My personal branches on my tree of life continue to grow and expand as I continue my life's journey. I water and prune and take joy in the shade of my tree of life. I continuously work hard to make sure it, like me, stays healthy.

BALANCE

"Every situation, properly perceived, becomes an opportunity to heal."

—*A Course in Miracles*

I *love* camping. Being surrounded by nature is where my bipolar disorder goes to sleep. It's just quiet. No bills to pay, phone or e-mail to answer. No TV, cars, home alarms, traffic or stores. *Nothing.* My body slows down. Like a battery running low, though, my mind takes longer to adjust. And then—ahh. I'm back where I belong. My breathing becomes easier with each inhalation of the cleanliness of nature (except when walking past latrines).

I've been going camping since I was in Camp Fire (Girl Scouts) at the ripe young age of 8-years-old. Not having to shower daily and getting to sleep outdoors in sleeping bags was really cool. I didn't realize until many, many years later (post-college) just how effective an environmental change could be in maintaining my inner balance or harmony.

I never understood why I loved packing for a camping trip and heading out of town, but dreaded returning back home to the city. I remember feeling stress return to my shoulders. It became hard to breathe, like I had asthma. I

245

got anxious, but I didn't know why. It happened every time we returned from a camping trip—and I hated it. I think my internal body went into shock and was trying to readjust itself to city life.

Balance has always been a part of my life, although until recently, I didn't realize how crucial it was to my being. There's the balance among work and play, alone time and time with my parents and friends. I definitely value my alone time. I think being an only child I have this engrained in me. If I don't get adequate "me" time, I get irritable. I've always been this way. I think having adequate alone time is necessary for my inner body to relax, like being in nature. I purposely slow things down and adjust my activities to my energy level. It's required time and patience, but I'm thankful I've learned what I need to operate most effectively and efficiently.

For me to be my best, I need adequate rest—nine hours of sleep with an hour nap daily, my morning prayer time, time to create and time to be with others, including walking Tigger every day.

My daily balance requires discipline and regularity. My daily activity cards help alleviate my anxiety I experience each morning. I listen to my body and try to pay attention to what I need. Sometimes it feels like I'm tending after a young child with the things I need, but I know I generally feel better when I take good care of myself.

I think the biggest lesson for me in trying to obtain daily balance is that there are days when things don't go according to plan or something that I want to do comes up out of the blue. So, if I schedule an evening out to see Michael Bublé in concert and don't get home until midnight, I know I'm going to have to pay the consequence the next day. I just don't know how severe or how long it's going to last.

BALANCE

I knew when the tickets were purchased for the Bublé concert that this was going to happen. I got an emotional hangover that absolutely wiped me out. Fortunately, I was able to sleep most of the next day and take it easy. I watched a movie at home, took Tigger on a walk, had some dinner, took my meds and read until I fell asleep.

I'm not hard on myself when I experience emotional hangovers. That particular one passed in two days, but it was totally worth it. I would do it again just to see and hear Michael in person. That was one fantastic concert!

And it's not just concerts that affect me, it's everything I choose to participate in. It also takes me a day to recuperate from giving "In Our Own Voice" presentations. The emotional and mental energy it takes me to prepare requires double the time to recover from it and return to being in balance.

These emotional hangovers have been occurring for several years. It took me a while to figure out what was going on and, more importantly, what I could do to fix them. I've talked to other people about emotional hangovers, but they don't experience them. I guess it's one of those bipolar symptoms specific to my case.

I'm thankful I have a flexible schedule where I can take a nap if I need to and where I'm given plenty of alone time each day. It's how I charge my battery.

So, whether the activity is fun or work-related or even errands, I exert a certain amount of energy. I don't know how long this will continue to be a symptom of my illness. But for now, I honor what I need—whether physical, mental, emotional or spiritual. Like taking care of a car, my personal maintenance is necessary so I can run at my optimum or best.

When things start breaking down, I try to address them as soon as possible so I can return to being in balance. I turn to reviewing my WRAP plan, talking to Pete, having a good cry or taking a long walk around the neighborhood to clear my head.

The one time my energy seems to maintain a pretty steady balance is when I'm camping. Something about being in nature and hearing the birds and running river nearby brings me to a state of steady calmness. It's where my nerves are quieted, the thoughts in my mind clear away and I feel an all-encompassing peacefulness.

Maybe this is why people like getting away to the mountains. It's certainly my place where I can be with God and where my bipolar, SAD, OCD and paranoia symptoms are hushed away by the gentle back-and-forth sweeping of tall pine trees. The shade cools my anger and I begin to talk to God. I still take my meds when I go camping, but I know it's the environment that I crave to return to each summer. Who knew that something I did 26 years ago would turn out to be such a saving grace?

And for the rest of the year? To keep my supply of nature going year round and keep me in balance, I have nature CDs, hot tub soaks, books that transport me to other places and times, a table-top fountain in my room, nature photos and a well-frequented bird bath in the back yard.

ROAD TO RECOVERY

"Problems do not go away. They must be worked through or else they remain, forever a barrier to the growth and development of the spirit."

—M. Scott Peck

My road to recovery is never-ending. Each day when I awake, I choose between wellness or succumbing to my illness. It's easier, much easier actually, to choose wellness when I'm feeling good. Oh, if only I could capture those moments, those days and bottle them up for when I'm having a really crummy day. I could sprinkle my "happy feelings" all over me and drench myself in them until I return to the me that I know and love.

There are times, I admit, when I'm so depressed and in such an absolutely rotten mood that even I can't stand to be around me. It's times like these when I try my hardest to take really good care of myself—physically, mentally, emotionally and spiritually. I make it my priority to pamper myself because, honestly, I know myself better than anyone else, and I usually know what I need. Sometimes it's inner-child Michelle taking care of adult Michelle. At other times, it's reversed—as if tending a young child.

I have acquired an abundance of wellness tools that I

use when I feel myself slipping out of wellness. Most of the things I do require minimal travel time. They also don't require a lot of money.

I just tap into my mood and listen to what I need. And if it so happens that I'm craving shopping, then I'll visit a local thrift store or consignment store and find something to pick up my mood. I feel good because I'm saving a ton of money and helping to recycle at the same time.

Getting quiet and listening to your inner voice will help you determine what works best to bring you back into balance. I think the biggest key is making time to figure out what tools work best. The question is how do you want to invest your time, energy and money? "I have what I need. I need what I have." That's one of my favorite quotes. There's such balance in this statement.

My past has definitely helped shape me into the person I am today. What occurred prior to my diagnosis and during the time I was hospitalized seven years ago is something that I'll never forget. It was very traumatic and for that reason I have "scared myself into wellness." I never want to get manic again or have to be hospitalized. While some of it was humorous, most of the time it scared me so much I thought I was in a horror movie with no director.

I can pull up these memories from my diagnosis at any time. Remembering the trauma keeps me well. Another thing that I contend with on a regular basis is my eating disorder. It's second in line after my bipolar disorder and it, too, is a mental illness. Stress is the thing that drives both illnesses. The more stress I'm under, the more control I need to have in my life. And if I don't, then my anorexic eating patterns burst through the surface.

To stay healthy, I really need to monitor my stress level. Most of the time things are fine and I don't think about stress at all. But when I have an argument with someone, or

I feel I'm being taken for granted or people aren't treating me with respect, then the eating disorder surfaces. Knowing what triggers it helps a lot. There is no cure for anorexia. I've been in remission for 23 years, meaning not having an episode or being hospitalized for it. It comes in waves and the severity and duration depends on the stressor.

I'll *never* forget my past. It's tattooed in my brain and occasionally a flashback comes up that reminds me of it. I've chosen to learn and grow from my life experiences and to look back for reference purposes. I try to keep to a minimum my dwelling on the past, but sometimes my horrendous flashbacks take over my brain. When I relive a horrible past experience, it sticks with me—sometimes for hours and sometimes for days. It's like a needle pricking my brain over and over at one particular scene or event from any age in my life. Something sets me off, a trigger, such as what a person says. I then spiral down and out-of-control–like riding a roller coaster in the dark without handlebars and not knowing what direction or speed my mood is going to take me.

Even with medication, I still experience these downward spirals, but they usually don't last long and I've gotten better at "catching" myself and redirecting my mood. I call it "thought stopping." I literally stop whatever negative thought or "monkey mind" chatter is overwhelming me and making me anxious. I'll physically make a change in order to turn my brain off. I'll go for a walk, call a friend, just do something completely different to stop myself from thinking about the negative thought.

Later on, either hours or sometimes days later, I'll go back and mentally revisit what it was that bothered me about the negative thought. I find I'm in a better frame of mind and can think logically about it and decide how to resolve it.

My crying spells come in waves. Even an anti-anxiety medication can only do so much. I'm very good at mentally beating up on myself and I will replay conversations in my head over and over, thinking things are horrible and that people don't care about me or my feelings.

I can't believe that seven years have gone by since my diagnosis of bipolar disorder. The more I think about it, I don't see my life as becoming more complicated (which implies stress to me); instead, it is "comfortably blessed." I define this by these areas in my life (in order of importance): God, family and friends, personal growth, physical/mental/emotional/spiritual health, significant other, fun/recreation, career, money, and physical environment/home.

It's a combination of these areas over the past seven years that has helped me redefine my life and who I am now. Yes, there are a lot of categories and it requires time and patience for me to achieve a comfortable level of inner and outer balance. But by doing this, I'm able to achieve peace and happiness.

Was God with me during my dark days and hospitalizations? You bet. It took me a long time to believe it. I thought at the time, why in the world would God put me through so much pain? I'm a good person. I must have done some bad shit to the nuns during my Catholic school years and now it's payback time.

I've learned to trust God more as the years passed by. He became the best friend who I could rely on for comfort and guidance. His voice is loud and clear and something else—loving. I knew I could trust this voice because I came to believe that everything happens for a reason—the good, the bad, and the ugly—and that God was by my side, through it all.

Hearing God's voice brought me inner peace and calmness. I had never had such a regular, strong connection with Him before. He is like a good cup of spiritual coffee to wake me up and get me headed in the right direction each day. Being stable on my medications, I knew I was safe to pursue conversations with Him. I didn't feel like God—not at all. And this was definitely a nice relief. Solving the world's problems, while a very noble deed, was extremely stressful.

I know, without a doubt, that one purpose of me being diagnosed with bipolar disorder is so that this book could be written. I never knew I was an author, but with God's help the words flowed onto page after page, like He was dictating a letter to me. It was an amazing feeling and I felt incredibly close to Him while writing *Bipolar No More*. But, it doesn't end here. I know there will be travel and meeting many interesting people and sharing and listening to others as they open up about their journeys with a mental illness.

I've never felt so connected to God as I have these past few years. He has brought people into my life to help me along my journey and to understand things in this "life school." There have been books, walks with friends and even crying to reach some level of understanding about things. But above all there's been His love and bringing others into my life to love me.

I see God all around me now, everyday. I feel very blessed. I look for His signs, whether they're through an eagle symbol or the opportunity to help someone. I recognize His hand in things by how I feel. Calm and relaxed—God led. Anxious and "monkey mind"—ego led.

The distinction is as easy for me to see as hearing an ambulance 50 yards away. Fortunately, my hearing is very good and I can usually prepare to change lanes early on, avoiding traffic complications. I let the ambulance pass, then return to my prior lane and continue on my journey. This would be a God-led reaction. A "monkey mind" reaction would be me having the radio blaring a favorite song and not hearing the siren until I look in my rear view mirror and see it quickly approaching from behind. I would go into "freak out" mode and pray for a space to open up in the other lane before the ambulance plows me over. Lack of preparation sums it up.

I'm very blessed that I've changed my ways of thinking to focus on God. It wasn't easy. No one told me how to retrain my brain to think about God. But now, I'm happy to say that about 85 percent of my mind is occupied by God thoughts and the other 15 percent is the "monkey mind" chatter. Sometimes it just won't go away, no matter how hard I try to pray, walk, talk or write it out. It's only then that I take my "chill pill," wait a few minutes, and return to being in the present moment.

I've recognized over the years, with practice and being tuned into my needs, that when I'm rested I'm in the "present moment." I think clearly, am relaxed and feel some level of control in my life. I have inner peace and it's easy to breathe. I just live moment to moment, appreciating all that God has given me–people and opportunities to make my life so blessed. And although stress may be in my life, I'm able to do a variety of healthy things to keep myself in balance.

Everything I do takes a toll on me physically and mentally. The intensity and duration of the activity—whether work or recreation—determines how long it will take me to recuperate and return to being in balance. When I don't get adequate rest (nine hours of sleep), or I push myself to do too many things, or I have a disagreement with a friend or family member, it's like a switch is flipped in my brain and "monkey mind" chatter resumes. It's like a talk radio station is turned on in my mind. "All talk, all the time." It's crazy making. It would be more tolerable if it were a Delilah talk show in my head, but no, it's more like nonsense talk, just filling up my brain. If I'm stressed about social situations in my life over which I have no control, or I'm worried about "the unknown," I'm prone to paranoia and anxiety. If these feelings overwhelm me, I become like a deer caught in headlights–I freeze, mentally. My brain blanks out and that's when I most need my "chill pills" to restore balance.

But there's one thing I keep "testing" as the years go by. My ability to go to the park with friends. I think the fact that I'm not just driving by, but am spending time there, that my anxiety level peaks. It becomes hard for me to breathe and I get paranoid as I take in my surroundings. I don't feel safe, not even in the presence of friends. I feel very vulnerable. Like at any moment someone could come along and start a conversation with me–just like Warren did. Harmless, at first. And the flashbacks return. At least I know this about myself and there's plenty of other public places I can go to with my friends.

● ● ●

I believe that God gives me little signs along my daily journey to help me. He gives me answers and brings opportunities and people into my life, even though sometimes I don't understand the outcome. I know it may not be what I would have chosen for myself, but I pray each day that with God's guidance I will come to understand His choices for me. With His help, I can move forward in love and accept that what is happening to me now is what's intended for me to experience to become a more faith-centered person.

When I do my AM prayer ritual, take a walk at the Nature Center, spend time tutoring the Albuquerque Reads kids, write, dance or be with people I care about, I feel God's presence the most. I feel alive and happy, and I wouldn't trade it for anything in the world.

A CONVERSATION
WITH MICHELLE

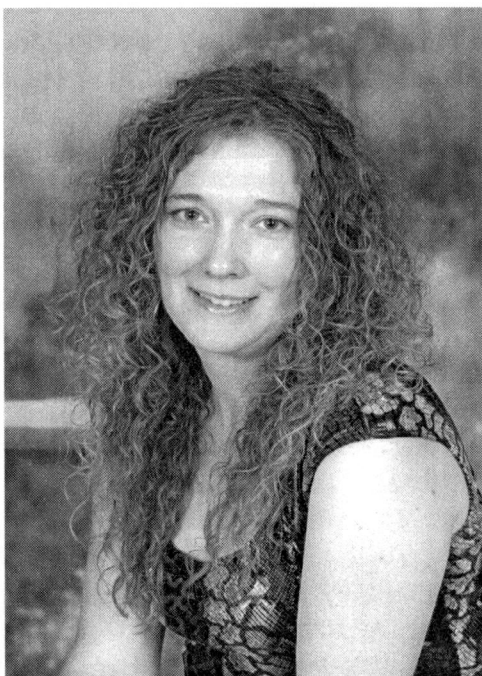

What does living in recovery mean or look like?

There is no specific "look" of a mentally ill person. We don't walk around with a stamp or birthmark on our foreheads. Basically, it means we're able to function in society just like a non-diagnosed person. It depends on our individual level of wellness how much we can take on. It's different for each person.

When I wake up, I rely on my daily activity cards to guide me through my day so I don't get overly anxious—my pattern for the past several years. I then know what I need to do each day. I try to balance work and play, alone time and time with others. Most days I'm able to achieve a balance and remain in the present moment. So for me, recovery means being in balance in all areas of my life: physical, emotional, mental and spiritual. I'm happy, relaxed and my thoughts are in the present moment.

Where did the idea for Bipolar No More *come from?*

When I was initially diagnosed seven years ago, the life I knew and loved vanished overnight. My life quickly became psychiatric visits, taking medications with names I couldn't pronounce and trying to find solace by talking to my parents. There were many questions that my doctors and parents couldn't answer, some of which I found in books–but there was still a huge void.

One day I just grabbed a plain spiral bound notebook and a pen (I wanted my thoughts to be permanent, no erasing allowed) and I started writing. As soon as I put my pen to paper it was like a race car speeding off. I couldn't write fast enough. I was in a stream of consciousness mode of writing. I wrote until my hand cramped or my brain ran out of thoughts. I call this style of writing "brain dumping," and it helped me work through my pain. Tears of anger, shame and disbelief trickled like raindrops on the pages, sometimes smearing the ink. But I didn't care. I wasn't writing to impress anyone. It felt like one huge, emotional construction project that I was jack hammering through. I was mad at God. And I wanted answers.

I never thought I'd be writing a book from all the note-books I filled over a six year period. The process was mainly therapeutic and it was one of my saving graces in my recovery process. A couple of years ago, I remember writing one day and the thought popped into my head, "I should write a book. I have enough material here." So, I did. I organized my stack of notebooks into chapters and began the process of writing *Bipolar No More*.

What was your goal in writing this book?

Initially it was to help me heal. But the more I wrote, the more it became an outreach for other consumers to use and help them in their recovery process. The theme that resonates through the book is hope—hope for everybody, no matter where they are in their recovery process, to know that recovery is possible. And I hope to inform and educate readers wherever they are in their path to recovery.

Why did you title it Bipolar No More?

That's an interesting question. It sounds as if I don't have the illness anymore. But I do. I want the title to be an attention grabber and I guess it worked. I think it sounds better than *Bipolar Still–Damn!* Hmm, maybe that'll be the sequel.

Bipolar No More has to do with stigma and not letting my illness run my life. As I frequently say, "I have bipolar disorder, it doesn't have me." Which means that, yes, I have this illness, but I'm choosing not to let it dictate my life any longer. I do what I need to in order to stay well—no different from diabetics who need to monitor their glucose levels throughout the day. I, too, need to monitor my moods and energy levels throughout the day. I do that, as in:

Taking daily medication, monitoring my stress level, getting adequate sleep, getting daily exercise, eating well and having daily interactions with people. I call those my "mental insulin." Reading my list might seem like a no-brainer. Don't let it fool you, though. It's not. It's a fine balance I am faced with maintaining every day.

The culprit is stress. The more of it I'm experiencing, the easier it is for me to get thrown off balance. Then I have the potential to experience an emotional flu that can easily zap me of all energy, which leaves me in a state where all I can do is just sleep it off until I'm in balance again.

Bipolar No More is about me taking control of my mental illness. I am not bipolar. I have bipolar disorder. That's a BIG difference. I have the illness, it doesn't have me. Probably my biggest pet peeve is when people say they're bipolar or ask if I am. I tell them I have bipolar disorder, but it's such a small, manageable part of my life now that I don't think about it that much. I did at the beginning, but I think it's smart to sort of move it out of the forefront as you become more well and balanced with time. I'm no longer ashamed to tell people I have bipolar disorder. It took me a long time, but it's very freeing to not be umbilically connected to a stigma-related word any longer.

What's the best advice you have for consumers?

I would say that each day is a new day. We always have the opportunity to start anew. Focus on where you want to be and take daily mini-steps to achieve your goals. Don't let your mental illness dictate your life. It's only a part of it—not all of it.

Whether diagnosed or not, we're all given a gift. Day by day, you choose the path you want to take. Is it God-driven or ego-driven? Remember, where you are today is a landmark for where you can be in a year's time. Pray for guidance and trust that God has placed you right where you are for a reason.

What are your plans now?

To catch my breath...and then to travel and promote my book. I love traveling—nationally and internationally. I look forward to speaking to people about my experiences of living with bipolar disorder. I look forward to connecting with others to help them learn how to live their life success-fully with the illness. I've got to be honest here. Having my book made into a movie would be really cool, too. I already know who I want to have play me!

I'll do regular Podcast seminars through my website.

I'd like to teach others how to write their memoirs, pos-sibly teaching on-line classes.

I'd love to be a guest speaker at a NAMI or DBSA na-tional convention. A year ago, I began writing an inspira-tional Christian novel that I entered in a writing contest. I won 3rd place. The first two chapters are complete. I plan to finish this book in the coming year.

What's your writing style? And how long did it take you to write this book?

Well, ever since my advertising days of writing on white paper with blue or black ink, I now opt for color—the brighter, the better. I went through almost one ream of pink bubblegum-colored paper and an assortment of colored gel pens to complete *Bipolar No More*. I began writing for one hour each morning with Tigger by my side after my cup of coffee in our family sunroom.

I wrote approximately three pages each day from Monday through Thursday. I took Fridays off. Being self-employed has its perks. Fridays began my three-day weekend where I would do fun things for me, such as taking in a movie, going to a museum, having lunch with a friend, doing whatever I felt like. It was my personal reward for a week of well-done work.

It took me about a year to complete this book. I think it actually took me longer to organize and read some of my notes then to actually sit at the computer and write. The tear-stained pages were definitely the most challenging, but not impossible to figure out.

How the chapters came to be formed is interesting. I literally put my pen to paper, and the words just flowed onto the pages. I never experienced writer's block, I just wrote from my heart. I was never anxious or worried what readers would say or think about me. And for all the pain and growth with this illness I went through over the past seven years, I never knew that I would write a book about my experiences to help others.

Talk about a surprise ending.

"It is good to have an end to journey toward but it is the journey that matters in the end."
—Ursula K. LeGuin

There may be days when you get up in the morning
And things aren't the way you had hoped they would be.
That's when you have to tell yourself that things will get better.
There are times when people disappoint you and let you down,
But those are the times when you must remind yourself
To trust your own judgments and opinions,
To keep your life focused on believing in yourself
And all that you are capable of.

There will be challenges to face and changes to make in your life,
And it is up to you to accept them.
Constantly keep yourself headed in the right direction for you.
It may not be easy at times, but in those times of struggle
You will find a stronger sense of who you are,
And you will also see yourself developing
Into the person you have always wanted to be.

Life is a journey through time, filled with many choices;
Each of us will experience life in our own special way.
So when the days come that are filled
With frustration and unexpected responsibilities,
Remember to believe in yourself and all you want your life to be,
Because the challenges and changes will only help you to find
The dreams that you know are meant to come true for you.

—Deanna Beisser

RESOURCES

The Depression and Bipolar Support Alliance (DBSA) www.dbsa.org. Contact your local DBSA office for information about free support groups.

The National Alliance on Mental Illness (NAMI) www.nami.org It has three free and invaluable education and support groups. Contact your local NAMI office for information on these programs:

Family-to-Family Class–Free, 12 week class open to family members of those with a mental illness.

Peer-to-Peer Class–Free, 10 week class open to consumers of mental health services.

Connections-Free, a weekly support group for consumers of mental health services.

Wellness and Recovery Action Plan (WRAP). For more information on this important advance directive go to www.mentalhealthrecovery.com

READING LIST

Over the past seven years, I have come across some very helpful books, some mental illness related and some not. When I come across a really good book, just like a really great shoe sale, I pass the information on to others. May these books inspire you and help you along your journey to recovery.

Ban Breathnach, Sarah. *Moving On: Creating Your House of Belonging With Simple Abundance* (Des Moines, Iowa: Meredith Books, 2006). When you've emotionally outgrown living where you're at, here is a thorough book that takes you step-by-step on your journey to prepare you to move forward with your life. Great quotes, too!

_____. *Something More: Excavating Your Authentic Self* (New York: Warner Bros Inc., 1998). When starting a journey, the author offers steps to guide you through life's tough times with grace, humor and insight.

Cameron, Julia *The Artist's Way: A Spiritual Path to Higher Creativity.* (New York: Penguin Putnam Inc., 1992) Tap into your creativity and learn about yourself. Highly recommend.

Carlson, Richard, Ph.D. *Don't Sweat the Small Stuff... and It's All Small Stuff* (New York: Hyperion, 1997). Start at the beginning or turn to a specific page. Whatever page you begin on, you'll get great advice.

Chodron, Pema. *When Things Fall Apart: Heart Advice for Difficult Times* (Shambhala Publications, Inc., 2005). Learn how to be compassionate when faced with emotional pain. Excellent read.

Dreamer, Oriah Mountain. *The Call: Discovering Why You Are Here* (New York/San Francisco: Harper, 2003). There's something within us all, our calling, that if we're open to hearing it and following it, it will change our lives.

Duke, Patty. *A Brilliant Madness: Living with Manic-Depressive Illness* (New York: Bantam Books, 1992). My introductory book to the world of bipolar disorder and mental illness. Given to me by a family member when I was first hospitalized.

Earley, Pete. *Crazy: A Father's Search Through America's Mental Health Madness* (New York: G.P. Putam's Sons, 2006). A father's search for psychiatric help for his grown son and what he encounters within the mental healthcare system as he seeks answers for his son and himself. Highly recommend.

Fisher, Carrie. *The Best Awful* (New York: Simon & Schuster Paperbacks, 2003). Novel of a woman diagnosed with manic-depression (bipolar disorder) and her struggles and triumphs as she goes in and out of psychiatric hospitals. Funny, touching and very real.

Fulghum, Robert. *All I Really Need To Know I Learned In Kindergarten: Uncommon Thoughts on Common Things* (New York: Ivy Books, 1988). Whatever your age, this book contains good advice on what really matters in life. Short chapters with great lessons–a modern Aesop's Fable.

Gill, Libby. *Traveling Hopefully: How To Lose Your Family Baggage And Jumpstart Your Life* (New York: St. Martin's Press, 2004). How to heal from your past and stay focused on moving forward. Helpful examples to jump start the life you want to have. Highly recommend.

Jamison, Kay Redfield. *An Unquiet Mind: A Memoir of Moods and Madness* (New York: Vintage Books, 1996). Jamison is a professor of psychiatry and someone who has bipolar disorder, and both perspectives are woven into her deeply moving account. Highly recommend.

Martin, Courney E. *Perfect Girls, Starving Daughters– The Frightening New Normalcy of Hating Your Body* (New York: The Free Press, 2007). An in-depth look at why, how and what drives women of all ages to develop eating disorders and what we can learn from them.

Meyer, Joyce. *Starting Your Day Right: Devotions for Each Morning of the Year* (New York: Faith Words, 2004). Short, daily inspirational messages from the Bible that can be read and applied to your life. (Flip side of book is called *Ending Your Day Right: Devotions for Each Evening of the Year*)

Miklowitz, David J., PhD. *The Bipolar Disorder Survival Guide: What You and Your Family Need to Know* (New York: The Guilford Press, 2002) Just the facts, please.

A great place for the newly diagnosed.

Mondimore, Francis Mark, M.D. *Bipolar Disorder: A Guide for Patients and Families* (Baltimore: Johns Hopkins University Press, 2006). A helpful resource by a psychiatrist with up-to-date information on the illness, its origins, diagnosis, treatment and recovery.

Mountain, Jane, M.D. *Beyond Bipolar: 7 Steps to Wellness* (Denver, CO: Chapter One Press, 2008). Focus is on hope and resiliency. Chapters are short, broken down in easy-to-read sections. Each chapter has questions at end for reflection. Highly recommend.

New American Bible (New York: Catholic Book Publishing Co., 1992). Easy-to-read translation. You can do search on topics in index. Recommended for any level Bible reader.

Picoult, Jodi. *Keeping Faith* (New York: HarperCollins Publishers, 1999). This novel is a quick read and will have you hooked on the first page. It incorporates accurate information about mental illness. Highly recommend.

St. James, Elaine. *Inner Simplicity: 100 Ways to Regain Peace and Nourish your Soul* (New York: Hyperion, 1995). Great advice on your journey to inner simplicity. Practical, easy-to-read with suggestions to make positive changes in your life. Read separately or accompanying *Simplify Your Life*.

_____. *Simplify Your Life: 100 Ways to Slow Down and Enjoy the Simple Things that Really Matter* (New York: Hyperion, 1994). A practical little book packed with great advice that you can implement in your life right now. Great to read during lunch or on an afternoon break.

Sacher, Ira M., M.D. *Regaining Your Self: Breaking Free From the Eating Disorder Identity: A Bold New Approach* (New York: Hyperion, 2007). Offers a message of hope for those willing to break free from the eating disorder cycle. Highly recommend.

Sacker, Ira M., M.D., Zimmer Marc A. Ph.D. *Dying To Be Thin: Understanding and Defeating Anorexia Nervosa and Bulimia—A Practical, Lifesaving Guide* (New York: Grand Central Publishing, 1987). How, when and where anorexics, bulimics and their family members can seek help. Focus is on understanding these illnesses and returning to healthy lifestyle. Highly recommend.

Seuss, Dr. *Oh, The Places You'll Go!* (New York: Random House 1990). Whatever your age, this book is meant for anyone who's starting a new journey in life. Indispensable.

Stout, Rev. Dr. James T., *Bipolar Disorder: Rebuilding Your Life* (California: Cypress House, 2002). Highly recommend for anyone wanting an empathetic account of living with bipolar disorder. Wide variety of topics, faith-based.

Whiffen, Valerie, Ph.D. *A Secret Sadness* (Oakland, CA: New Harbinger Publications, Inc., 2006) An insightful book for women. Depression as you've never seen it before.

NEED A SPEAKER?

Michelle Holtby, author of *Bipolar No More*, is available for speaking engagements. Whether the setting is informal or formal, she's available to talk about a variety of topics she discusses in her book, including ways to heal the body, soul and mind. She specializes in tailoring presentations to meet your specific needs.

Filled with insight, hope and humor her message is sure to make your event memorable. Her true stories will have you relating to her in no time. She takes the mystery out of the bipolar disorder story while answering common and not so common questions.

Her past audiences have included psychiatric inpatients, college students, staff and faculty, nursing students and churches. Whether the audience is small or large, her ability to tell her story is compelling. Her personable, caring manner attracts people from all walks of life.

Her ability to shine a bright light of hope on mental illness is something so few have addressed. Her ease with connecting with the audience will leave them looking at mental illness from a different perspective–that recovery is possible, no matter where you are in your diagnosis stage. She also shares invaluable mental wellness tools that the audience can use immediately, whether they have bipolar disorder or not.

Michelle is available for podcasts or live speaking engagements. Her life experiences living with bipolar disorder will open your eyes to the world of mental illness leaving you with an optimistic view of hope and recovery about this mysterious and often misunderstood illness.

Learn more at: <u>bipolarnomore.com</u>

Printed in the United States
205314BV00001B/151/P

9 781432 731380